&EPA

Cross-Connection
Control Manual

United States
Environmental Protection Agency
Office of Water
Office of Ground Water and Drinking Water

First Printing 1973
Reprinted 1974, 1975
Revised 1989
Reprinted 1995
Technical Corrections 2003

Preface

Plumbing cross-connections, which are defined as actual or potential connections between a potable and nonpotable water supply, constitute a serious public health hazard. There are numerous, well-documented cases where cross-connections have been responsible for contamination of drinking water, and have resulted in the spread of disease. The problem is a dynamic one, because piping systems are continually being installed, altered, or extended.

Control of cross-connections is possible, but only through thorough knowledge and vigilance. Education is essential, for even those who are experienced in piping installations fail to recognize cross-connection possibilities and dangers. All municipalities with public water supply systems should have cross-connection control programs. Those responsible for institutional or private water supplies should also be familiar with the dangers of cross-connections and should exercise careful surveillance of their systems.

This *Cross-Connection Control Manual* has been designed as a tool for health officials, water-works personnel, plumbers, and any others involved directly or indirectly in water supply distribution systems. It is intended to be used for educational, administrative, and technical reference in conducting cross-connection control programs. This manual is a revision of an earlier book entitled *Water Supply and Plumbing Cross-Connections* (PHS Publication Number 957), which was produced under the direction of Floyd B. Taylor by Marvin T. Skodje, who wrote the text and designed the illustrations.

Many of the original illustrations and text have been retained in this edition. Previous revisions were done by Peter C. Karalekas, Jr. with guidance from Roger D. Lee incorporating suggestions made by the staff of the EPA Water Supply Division, other governmental agencies, and interested individuals.

This 3rd edition was produced as a result of an updated need for cross-connection control reference material reflecting an increase in cross-connection control activity throughout the United States. It has been revised and re-issued reflecting a demand for its use, together with requests for a document that covers the broad spectrum of cross-connection control from both the basic hydraulic concepts through the inclusion of a sample program that can be a guide for a program at the municipal level. New backflow devices have been included in this revision that are now being produced by manufacturers reflecting the needs of the market. Updated actual cross-connection case histories have been added containing graphic schematic illustrations showing how the incidents occurred and how cross-connection control practices could be applied to eliminate future re-occurrence. A more detailed explanation of cross-connection control "containment" practice has been included together with the use for "internal backflow protective devices" and "fixture outlet protection".

This 1989 edition was prepared by Howard D. Hendrickson, PE, vice president of Water Service Consultants, with assistance from Peter C. Karalekas, Jr. of Region 1, EPA, Boston.

This latest (2003) edition has technical corrections provided by Howard D. Hendrickson, P.E., showing updates on pages iv, 18, 23, 30, 31, and 32.

Contents

An AWWA Statement of Policy on Public Water Supply Matters.

Cross Connections

Adopted by the Board of Directors Jan. 26, 1970, revised June 24, 1979, reaffirmed June 10, 1984 and revised Jan. 28, 1990 and Jan. 21, 2001.

The American Water Works Association (AWWA) recognizes water purveyors have the responsibility to supply potable water to their customers. In the exercise of this responsibility, water purveyors or other responsible authorities must implement, administer, and maintain ongoing backflow prevention and cross-connection control programs to protect public water systems from the hazards originating on the premises of their customers and from temporary connections that may impair or alter the water in the public water systems. The return of any water to the public water system after the water has been used for any purpose on the customer's premises or within the customer's piping system is unacceptable and opposed by AWWA.

The water purveyor shall assure that effective backflow prevention measures commensurate with the degree of hazard, are implemented to ensure continual protection of the water in the public water distribution system. Customers, together with other authorities are responsible for preventing contamination of the private plumbing system under their control and the associated protection of the public water system.

If appropriate back-flow prevention measures have not been taken, the water purveyor shall take or cause to be taken necessary measures to ensure that the public water distribution system is protected from any actual or potential backflow hazard. Such action would include the testing, installation, and continual assurance of proper operation and installation of backflow-prevention assemblies, devices, and methods commensurate with the degree of hazard at the service connection or at the point of cross connection or both. If these actions are not taken, water service shall ultimately be eliminated.

To reduce the risk private plumbing systems pose to the public water distribution system, the water purveyor's backflow prevention program should include public education regarding the hazards backflow presents to the safety of drinking water and should include coordination with the cross connection efforts of local authorities, particularly health and plumbing officials. In areas lacking a health or plumbing enforcement agency, the water purveyor should additionally promote the health and safety of private plumbing systems to protect its customers from the hazards of backflow.

Chapter One

Purpose and Scope

Public health officials have long been concerned about cross-connections and backflow connections in plumbing systems and in public drinking water supply distribution systems. Such cross-connections, which make possible the contamination of potable water, are ever-present dangers. One example of what can happen is an epidemic that occurred in Chicago in 1933. Old, defective, and improperly designed plumbing and fixtures permitted the contamination of drinking water. As a result, 1,409 persons contracted amebic dysentery; there were 98 deaths. This epidemic, and others resulting from contamination introduced into a water supply through improper plumbing, made clear the responsibility of public health officials and water purveyors for exercising control over public water distribution systems and all plumbing systems connected to them. This responsibility includes advising and instructing plumbing installers in the recognition and elimination of cross-connections.

Cross-connections are the links through which it is possible for contaminating materials to enter a potable water supply. The contaminant enters the potable water system when the pressure of the polluted source exceeds the pressure of the potable source. The action may be called backsiphonage or backflow. Essentially it is reversal of the hydraulic gradient that can be produced by a variety of circumstances.

It might be assumed that steps for detecting and eliminating cross-connections would be elementary and obvious. Actually, cross-connections may appear in many subtle forms and in unsuspected places. Reversal of pressure in the water may be freakish and unpredictable. The probability of contamination of drinking water through a cross-connection occurring within a single plumbing system may seem remote; but, considering the multitude of similar systems, the probability is great.

Why do such cross-connections exist?

First, plumbing is frequently installed by persons who are unaware of the inherent dangers of cross-connections. Second, such connections are made as a simple matter of convenience without regard to the dangerous situation that might be created. And, third, they are made with reliance on inadequate protection such as a single valve or other mechanical device.

To combat the dangers of cross-connections and backflow connections, education in their recognition and prevention is needed. First, plumbing installers must know that hydraulic and pollutional factors may combine to produce a sanitary hazard if a cross-connection is present. Second, they must realize that there are available reliable and simple standard backflow prevention devices and methods that may be substituted for the convenient but dangerous direct connection. And third, it should be made clear to all that the hazards resulting from direct connections greatly outweigh the convenience gained. This manual does not describe all the cross-connections possible in piping systems. It does attempt to reduce the subject to a statement of the principles involved and to make it clear to the reader that such installations are potentially dangerous. The primary purpose is to define, describe, and illustrate typical cross-connections and to suggest simple methods and devices by which they may be eliminated without interfering with the functions of plumbing or water supply distribution systems.

Chapter Two

Public Health Significance of Cross-Connections

Human Blood in the Water System

Public health officials have long been aware of the impact that cross-connections play as a threat to the public health. Because plumbing defects are so frequent and the opportunity for contaminants to invade the public drinking water through cross-connections are so general, enteric illnesses caused by drinking water may occur at most any location and at any time.

The following documented cases of cross-connection problems illustrate and emphasize how actual cross-connections have compromised the water quality and the public health.

Health Department officials cut off the water supply to a funeral home located in a large southern city, after it was determined that human blood had contaminated the fresh water supply. City water and plumbing officials said that they did not think that the blood contamination had spread beyond the building, however, inspectors were sent into the neighborhood to check for possible contamination. The chief plumbing inspector had received a telephone call advising that blood was coming from drinking fountains within the building. Plumbing and county health department inspectors went to the scene and found evidence that the blood had been circulating in the water system within the building. They immediately ordered the building cut off from the water system at the meter.

Investigation revealed that the funeral home had been using a hydraulic aspirator to drain fluids from the bodies of human "remains" as part of the embalming process. The aspirator directly connected to the water supply system at a faucet outlet located on a sink in the "preparation" (embalming) room. Water flow through the aspirator created suction that was utilized to draw body fluids through a hose and needle attached to the suction side of the aspirator.

The contamination of the funeral home potable water supply was caused by a combination of low water pressure in conjunction with the simultaneous use of the aspirator. Instead of the body fluids flowing into the sanitary drain, they were drawn in the opposite direction—into the potable water supply of the funeral home!

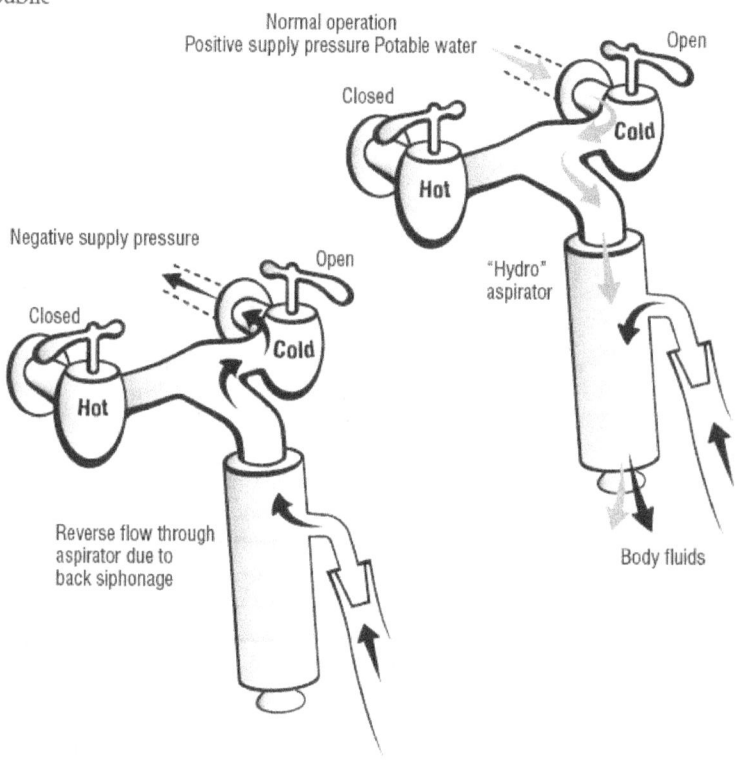

Normal operation
Positive supply pressure Potable water
Open
Closed
Cold
Hot
"Hydro" aspirator

Negative supply pressure
Open
Closed
Cold
Hot

Reverse flow through aspirator due to back siphonage

Body fluids

Burned in the Shower

A resident of a small town in Alabama, jumped in the shower at 5 a.m. one morning in October, 1986, and when he got out his body was covered with tiny blisters. "The more I rubbed it, the worse it got," the 60 year old resident said. "It looked like someone took a blow torch and singed me."

He and several other residents received medical treatment at the emergency room of the local hospital after the water system was contaminated with sodium hydroxide, a strong caustic solution.

Other residents claimed that, "It (the water) bubbled up and looked like Alka Seltzer. I stuck my hand under the faucet and some blisters came up."

One neighbor's head was covered with blisters after she washed her hair and others complained of burned throats or mouths after drinking the water.

The incident began after an 8-inch water main, that fed the town, broke and was repaired. While repairing the water main, one workman suffered leg burns from a chemical in the water and required medical treatment. Measurements of the ph of the water were as high as 13 in some sections of the pipe.

Investigation into the cause of the problem led to a possible source of the contamination from a nearby chemical company that distributes chemicals such as sodium hydroxide. The sodium hydroxide is brought to the plant in liquid form in bulk tanker trucks and is transferred to a holding tank and then pumped into 55 gallon drums. When the water main broke, a truck driver was adding the water from the bottom of the tank truck instead of the top, and sodium hydroxide back-siphoned into the water main.

Heating System Anti-Freeze into Potable Water

Bangor Maine Water Department employees discovered poisonous antifreeze in a homeowner's heating system and water supply in November, 1981. The incident occurred when they shut off 'the service line to the home to make repairs. With the flow of water to the house cut off, pressure in the lines in the house dropped and the anti-freeze, placed in the heating system to prevent freeze-up of an unused hot water heating system, drained out of the heating system into house water lines, and flowed out to the street. If it had not been noticed, it would have entered the homeowner's drinking water when the water pressure was restored.

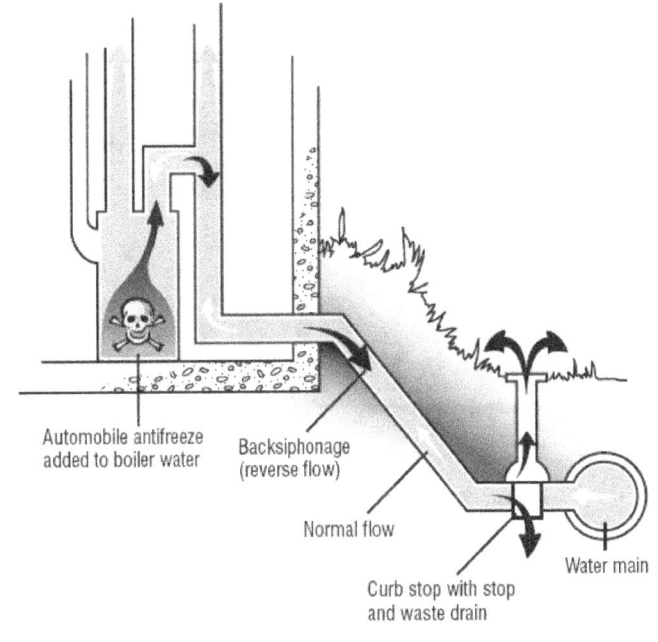

Automobile antifreeze added to boiler water

Backsiphonage (reverse flow)

Normal flow

Water main

Curb stop with stop and waste drain

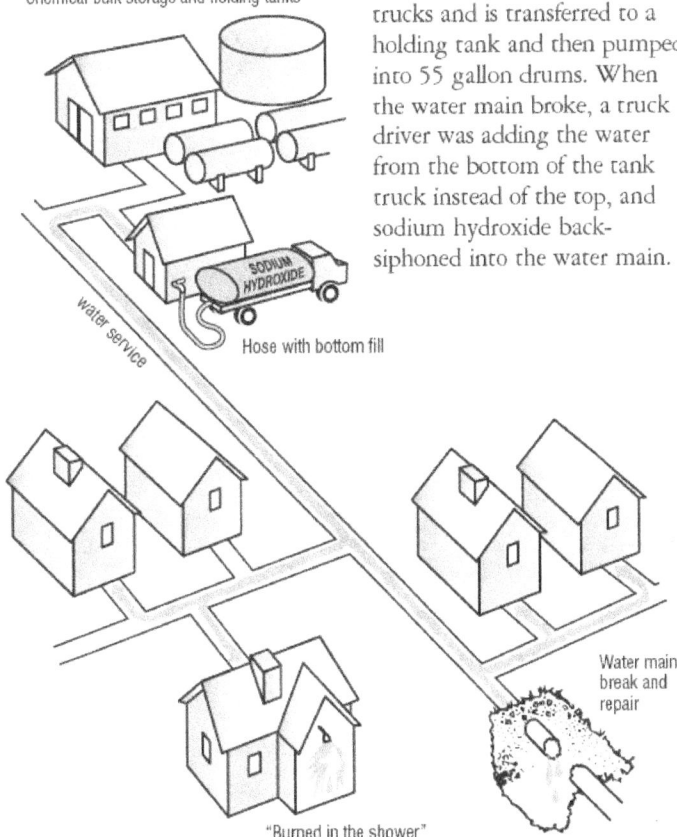

Chemical bulk storage and holding tanks

SODIUM HYDROXIDE

Water service

Hose with bottom fill

Water main break and repair

"Burned in the shower"

Salty Drinks

In January, 1981, a nationally known fast food restaurant located in southeastern United States, complained to the water department that all their soft drinks were being rejected by their customers as tasting "salty." This included soda fountain beverages, coffee, orange juice, etc. An investigation revealed that an adjacent water customer complained of salty water occurring simultaneously with the restaurant incident. This second complaint came from a water front ship repair facility that was also being served by the same water main lateral. The (investigation centered on the ship repair facility and revealed the following:

• A backflow preventer that had been installed on the service line to the shipyard had frozen and had been replaced with a spool piece sleeve.

• The shipyard fire protection system utilized sea water that was pumped by both electric and diesel driven pumps.

• The pumps were primed by potable city water.

With the potable priming line left open and the pumps maintaining pressure in the fire lines, raw salt water was pumped through the priming lines, through the spool sleeve piece, to the ship repair facility and the restaurant.

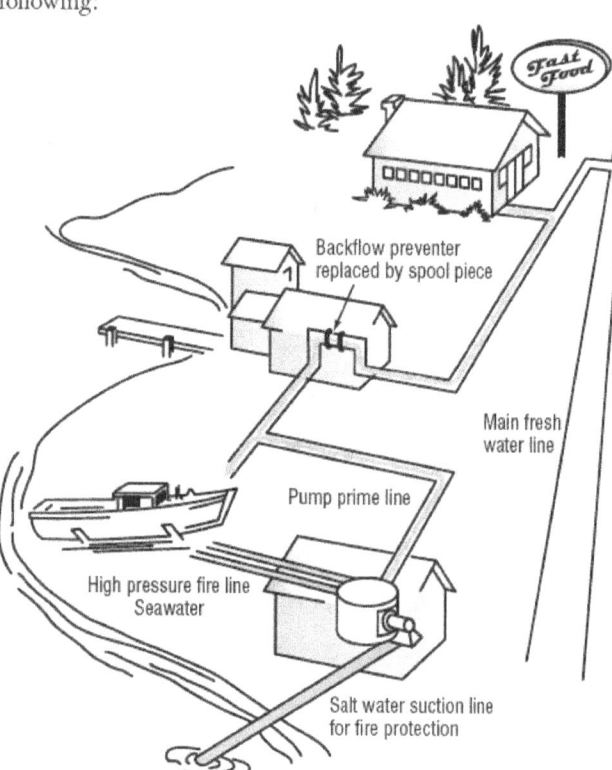

Backflow preventer replaced by spool piece

Main fresh water line

Pump prime line

High pressure fire line Seawater

Salt water suction line for fire protection

Paraquat in the Water System

"Yellow gushy stuff" poured from some of the faucets in a small town in Maryland, and the State of Maryland placed a ban on drinking the water supply. Residents were warned not to use the water for cooking, bathing, drinking or any other purpose except for flushing toilets.

The incident drew widespread attention and made the local newspapers. In addition to being the lead story on the ABC news affiliate in Washington, D.C. and virtually all the Washington/Baltimore newspapers that evening. The news media contended that lethal pesticides may have contaminated the water supply and among the contaminants was paraquat, a powerful agricultural herbicide.

The investigation disclosed that the water pressure in the town water mains was temporarily reduced due to a water pump failure in the town water supply pumping system. Coincidentally, a gate valve between a herbicide chemical holding tank and the town

water supply piping had been left open. A lethal cross-connection had been created that permitted the herbicide to flow into the potable water supply system. Upon restoration of water pressure, the herbicides flowed into the many faucets and outlets on the town water distribution system.

This cross-connection created a needless and costly event that fortunately did not result in serious illness or loss of life. Door-to-door public notification, extensive flushing, water sample analysis, emergency arrangements to provide temporary potable water from tanker trucks, all contributed to an expensive and unnecessary town burden.

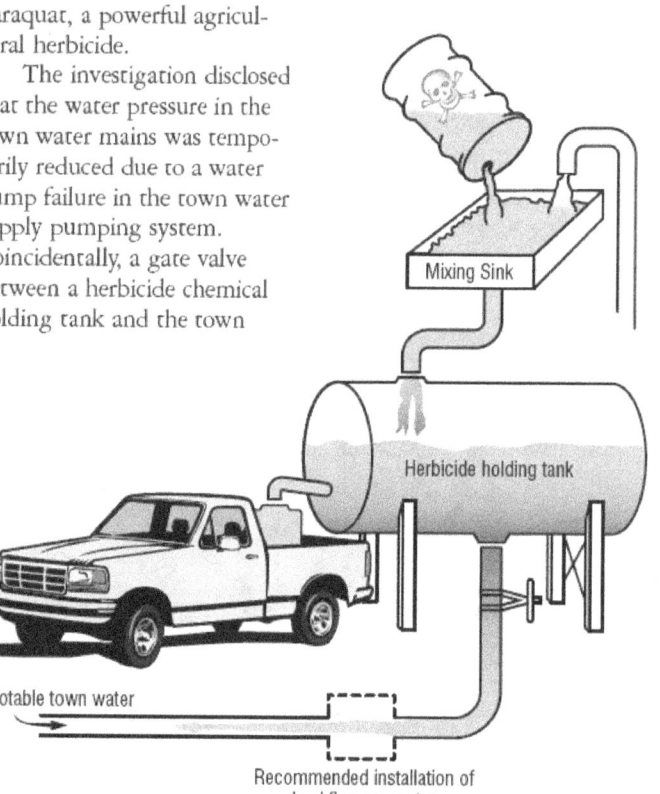

Mixing Sink

Herbicide holding tank

Potable town water

Recommended installation of backflow preventer

Propane Gas in the Water Mains

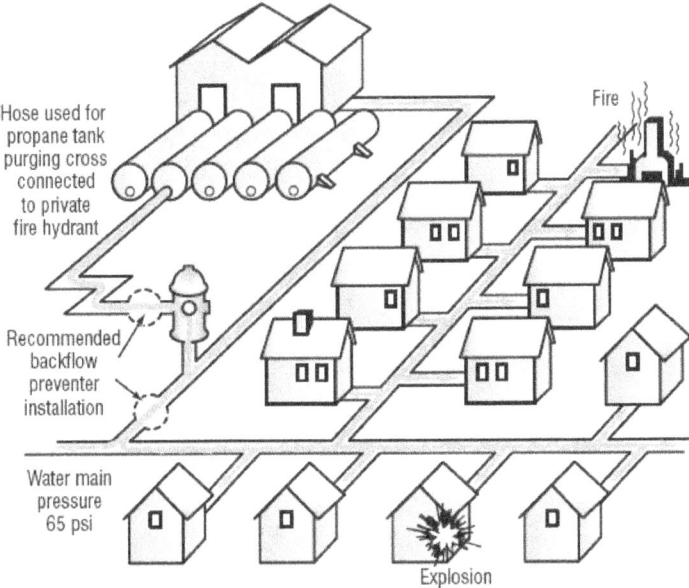

Hose used for propane tank purging cross connected to private fire hydrant

Fire

Recommended backflow preventer installation

Water main pressure 65 psi

Explosion

Hundreds of people were evacuated from their homes and businesses on an August afternoon in a town in Connecticut in 1982 as a result of propane entering the city water supply system. Fires were reported in two homes and the town water supply was contaminated. One five-room residence was gutted by a blaze resulting from propane gas "bubbling and hissing" from a bathroom toilet and in another home a washing machine explosion blew a woman against a wall. Residents throughout the area reported hissing, bubbling noises, coming from washing machines, sinks and toilets. Faucets sputtered out small streams of water mixed with gas and residents in the area were asked to evacuate their homes.

This near-disaster occurred in one, 30,000 gallon capacity liquid propane tank when the gas company initiated immedi-

ate repair procedures. To start the repair, the tank was "purged" of residual propane by using water from one of two private fire hydrants located on the property. Water purging is the preferred method of purging over the use of carbon dioxide since it is more positive and will float out any sludge as well as any gas vapors. The "purging" consisted of hooking up a hose to one of the private fire hydrants located on the property and initiating flushing procedures.

Since the vapor pressure of the propane residual in the tank was 85 to 90 psi., and the water pressure was only 65 to 70 psi., propane gas backpressure backflowed into the water main. It was estimated that the gas flowed into the water mains for about 20 minutes and that about 2,000 cubic feet of gas was involved. This was approximately enough gas to fill one mile of an 8-inch water main.

Chlordane and Heptachlor at the Housing Authority

The services to seventy five apartments housing approximately three hundred people were contaminated with chlordane and heptachlor in a city in Pennsylvania, in December, 1980. The insecticides entered the water supply system while an exterminating company was applying them as a preventative measure against termites. While the pesticide contractor was mixing the chemicals in a tank truck with water from a garden hose coming from one of the apartments, a workman was cutting into a 6-inch main line to install a gate valve. The end of the garden hose was submerged in the tank containing the pesticides, and at the same time, the water to the area was shut off and the lines being drained prior to the installation

of the gate valve. When the workman cut the 6-inch line, water started to drain out of the cut, thereby setting up a backsiphonage condition. As a result, the chemicals were siphoned out of the truck, through the garden hose, and into the system, contaminating the seventy five apartments.

Repeated efforts to clean and flush the lines were not satisfactory and it was finally decided to replace the water line and all the plumbing that was affected. There were no reports of illness, but residents of the housing authority were told not to use any tap water for any purpose and they were given water that was trucked into the area by volunteer fire department personnel. They were without their normal water supply for 27 days.

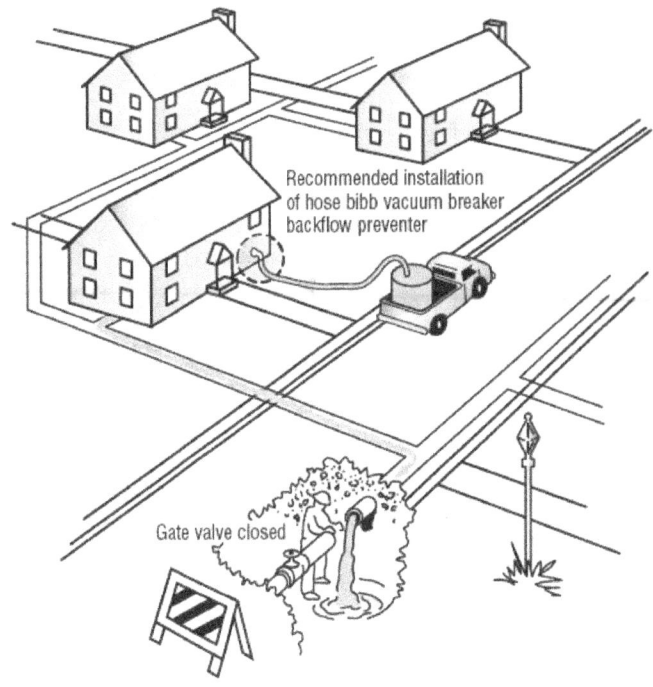

Recommended installation of hose bibb vacuum breaker backflow preventer

Gate valve closed

Boiler Water Enters High School Drinking Water

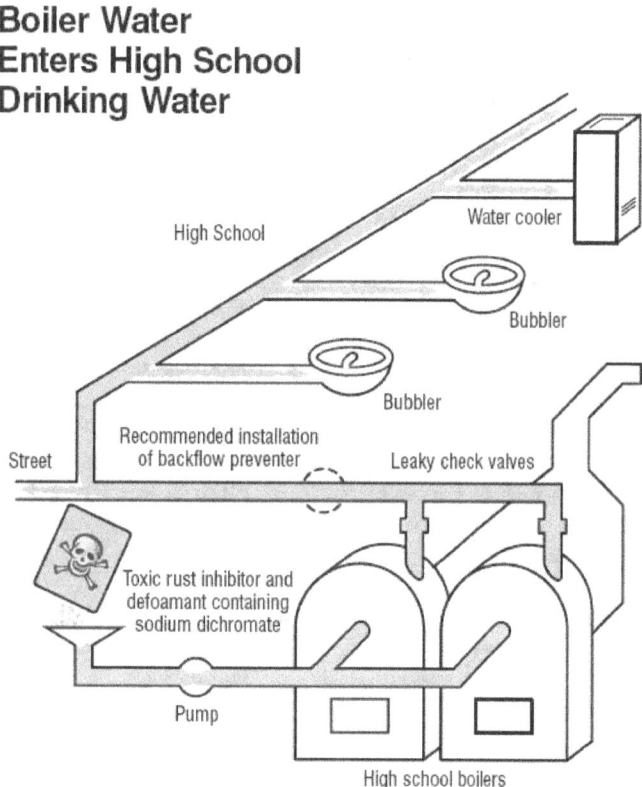

High School

Water cooler

Bubbler

Bubbler

Recommended installation of backflow preventer

Street

Leaky check valves

Toxic rust inhibitor and defoamant containing sodium dichromate

Pump

High school boilers

A high school in New Mexico, was closed for several days in June 1984 when a home economics teacher noticed the water in the potable system was yellow. City chemists determined that samples taken contained levels of chromium as high as 700 parts per million, "astronomically higher than the accepted levels of .05 parts per million." The head chemist said that it was miraculous that no one was seriously injured or killed by the high levels of chromium. The chemical was identified as sodium dichromate, a toxic form of chromium used in heating system boilers to inhibit corrosion of the metal parts.

No students or faculty were known to have consumed any of the water; however, area physicians and hospitals advised that if anyone had consumed those high levels of chromium, the symptoms would be nausea, diarrhea, and burning of the mouth and throat. Fortunately, the home economics teacher, who first saw the discolored water before school started, immediately covered all water fountains with towels so that no one would drink the water.

Investigation disclosed that chromium used in the heating system boilers to inhibit corrosion of metal parts entered the potable water supply system as a result of backflow through leaking check valves on the boiler feed lines.

Pesticide in Drinking Water

A pesticide contaminated a North Carolina water system in April, 1986, prompting the town to warn residents of 23 households not to drink the water. The residents in the affected area were supplied drinking water from a tank truck parked in the parking lot of a downtown office building until the condition could be cleared up. Residents complained of foul smelling water but there were no reports of illness from ingesting the water that had been contaminated with a pesticide containing chlordane and heptachlor.

Authorities stated that the problem occurred when a water main broke at the same time that a pest control service was filling a pesticide truck with water. The reduction in pressure caused the pesticide from inside the tank to be sucked into the building's water main. The pesticide contaminated the potable water supply of the office building and neighborhood area.

Car Wash Water in the Water Main Street

This car wash cross-connection and backpressure incident, which occurred in February, 1979, in the state of Washington, resulted in backflow chemical contamination of approximately 100 square blocks of water mains. Prompt response by the water department prevented a potentially hazardous water quality degradation problem without a recorded case of illness.

Numerous complaints of grey-green and "slippery" water were received by the water department coming from the same general area of town. A sample brought to the water department by a customer confirmed the reported problem and preliminary analysis indicated contamination with what appeared to be a detergent solution. While emergency crews initiated flushing operations, further investigation within the contaminated area signaled the problem was probably caused by a car wash,

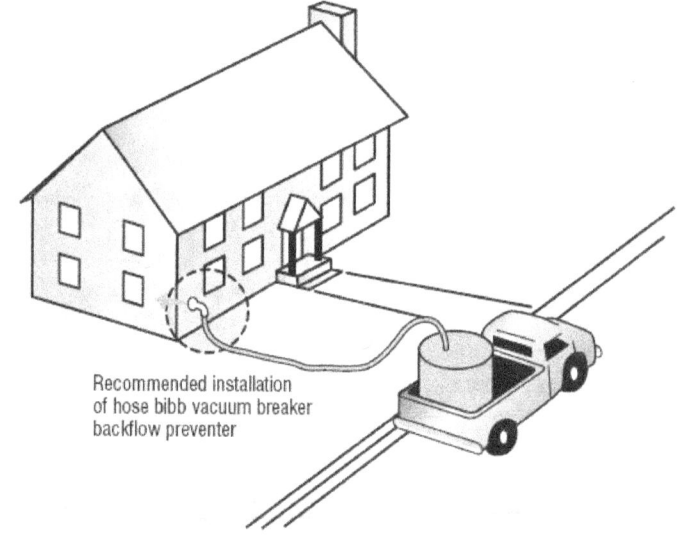

Recommended installation of hose bibb vacuum breaker backflow preventer

or laundry, based upon the soapy nature of the contaminant. The source was quickly narrowed down to a car wash and the proprietor was extremely cooperative in admitting to the problem and explaining how it had occurred. The circumstances leading up to the incident were as follows:

• On Saturday, February 10, 1979, a high pressure pump broke down at the car wash. This pump recycled reclaimed wash and rinse water and pumped it to the initial scrubbers of the car wash. No potable plumbing connection is normally made to the car wash's scrubber system.

• After the pump broke down, the car wash owner was able to continue operation by connecting a 2-inch hose section temporarily between the potable supply within the car wash, and the scrubber cycle piping.

• On Monday, February 12, 1979, the owner repaired the high pressure pump and resumed normal car wash operations. The 2-inch hose connection (cross-connection) was not removed!

• Because of the cross-connection, the newly repaired high pressure pump promptly pumped a large quantity of the reclaimed wash/rinse water out of the car wash and into a 12-inch water main in the street. This in turn was delivered to the many residences and commercial establishments connected to the water main.

Within 24 hours of the incident, the owner of the car wash had installed a 2-inch reduced pressure principle backflow preventer on his water service and all car wash establishments in Seattle that used a wash water reclaim system were notified of the state requirement for backflow prevention.

Shipyard Backflow Contamination

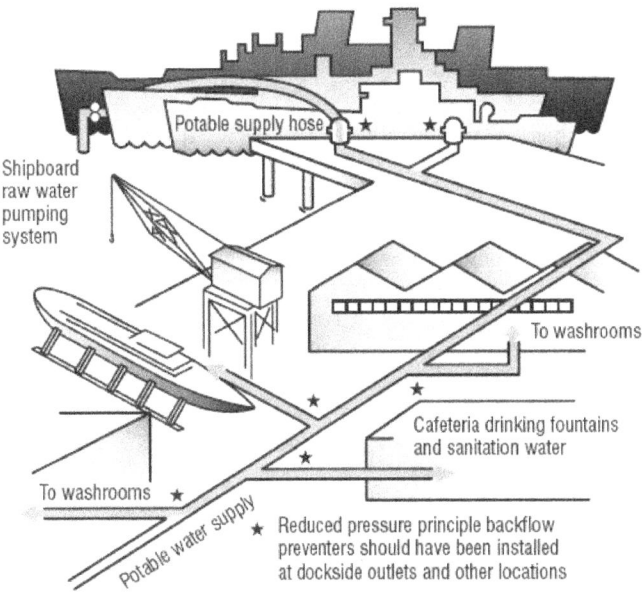

★ Reduced pressure principle backflow preventers should have been installed at dockside outlets and other locations

Water fountains at an East Coast Shipyard were posted "No Drinking" as workers flushed the water lines to eliminate raw river water that had entered the shipyard following contamination from incorrectly connected water lines between ships at the pier and the shipyard. Some third shift employees drank the water before the pollution was discovered and later complained of stomach cramps and diarrhea.

The cause of the problem was a direct cross-connection between the on-board salt water fire protection water system and the fresh water connected to one of the ships at the dock. While the shipyard had been aware of the need for backflow protection at the dockside tie up area, the device had not been delivered and installed prior to the time of the incident. As a result, the salt water on-board fire protection system, being at a greater pressure than the potable supply, forced the salt water, through backpressure, into the shipyard potable supply.

Fortunately, a small demand for potable water at the time of the incident prevented widespread pollution in the shipyard and the surrounding areas.

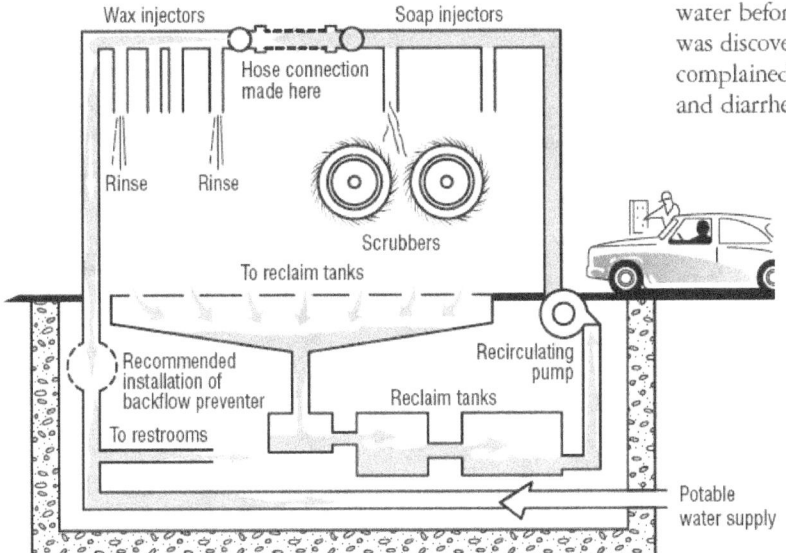

Chlordane in the Water Main

In October, 1979, approximately three gallons of chlordane, a highly toxic insecticide, was sucked back (back-siphoned) into the water system of a residential area of a good sized eastern city. Residents complained that the water "looked milky, felt greasy, foamed and smelled," and as one woman put it, "It was similar to a combination of kerosene and Black Flag pesticide."

The problem developed while water department personnel were repairing a water main. A professional exterminator, meanwhile, was treating a nearby home with chlordane for termite elimination. The workman for the exterminator company left one end of a garden hose that was connected to an outside hose bibb tap in a barrel of diluted pesticide. During the water service interruption, the chlordane solution was back-siphoned from the barrel through the house and into the water mains.

Following numerous complaints, the water department undertook an extensive program of flushing of the water mains and hand delivered letters telling residents to flush their lines for four hours before using the water. Until the water lines were clear of the contaminant, water was hand-hauled into homes, and people went out of their homes for showers, meals and every other activity involving potable water. Fortunately, due to the obvious bad taste, odor and color of the contaminated water, no one consumed a sufficient quantity to endanger health.

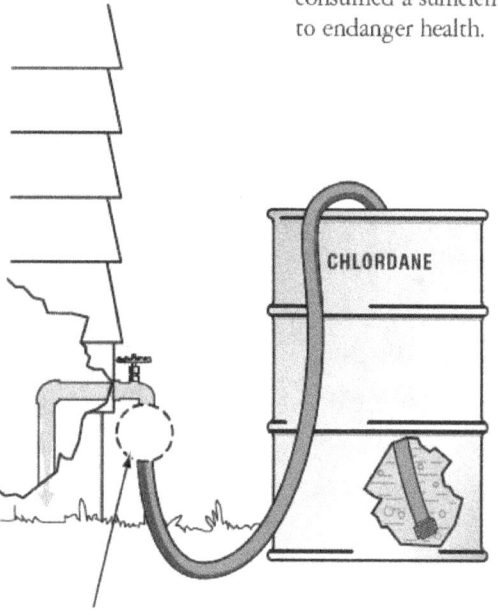

Recommended installation of hose bibb vacuum breaker backflow preventer

Hexavalent Chromium in Drinking Water

In July, 1982, a well meaning maintenance mechanic, in attempting to correct a fogging lens in an overcooled laser machine, installed a tempering valve in the laser cooling line, and inadvertently set the stage for a backpressure backflow incident that resulted in hexavalent chromium contaminating the potable water of a large electronic manufacturing company in Massachusetts employing 9,000 people. Quantities of 50 parts per million hexavalent chromium were found in the drinking water which is sufficient to cause severe vomiting, diarrhea, and intestinal sickness. Maintenance crews working during the plant shutdown were able to eliminate the cross-connection and thoroughly flush the potable water system, thereby preventing a serious health hazard from occurring.

The incident occurred as follows:

• Laser machine lenses were kept cool by circulating chilled water that came from a large refrigeration chiller. The water used in the chiller was treated with hexavalent chromium, a chemical additive used as an anticorrosive agent and an algicide. As a result, the chilled water presented a toxic, non-potable substance unfit for human consumption but very

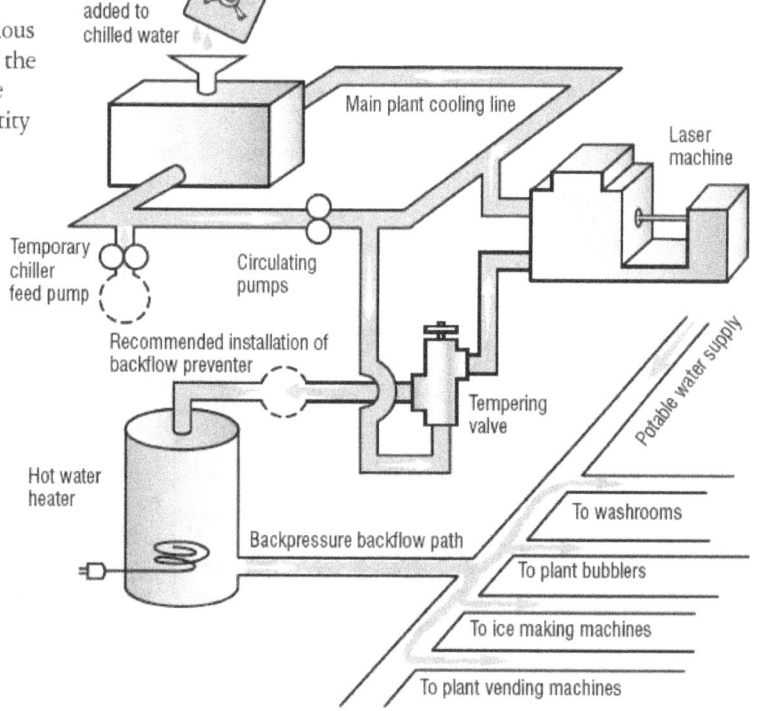

Employee Health Problems due to Cross-Connection

acceptable for industrial process water. No health hazard was present as long as the piping was identified, kept separate from potable drinking water lines, and not cross-connected to the potable water supply.

• A maintenance mechanic correctly reasoned that by adding a tempering valve to the chilled water line, he could heat up the water a bit and eliminate fogging of the laser lenses resulting from the chilled water being too cold. The problem with the installation of the tempering valve was that a direct cross-connection had been inadvertently made between the toxic chilled water and the potable drinking water line!

• Periodic maintenance to the chiller system was performed in the summer, requiring that an alternate chiller feed pump be temporarily installed. This replacement pump had an outlet pressure of 150 psi, and promptly established an imbalance of pressure at the tempering valve, thereby over-pressurizing the 60 psi, potable supply. Backpressure backflow resulted and pushed the toxic chilled water from the water heater and then into the plant's potable drinking water supply. Yellowish green water started pouring out of the drinking fountains, the washroom, and all potable outlets.

A cross-connection incident occurring in a modern seven-story office building located in a large city in New Hampshire, in March, 1980, resulted in numerous cases of nausea, diarrhea, loss of time and employee complaints as to the poor quality of the water.

On Saturday, March 1, 1980, a large fire occurred two blocks away from a seven-story office building in this large New Hampshire city. On Sunday, March 2, 1980, the maintenance crew of the office building arrived to perform the weekly cleaning, and after drinking the water from the drinking fountains, and sampling the coffee from the coffee machines, noticed that the water smelled rubbery and had a strong bitter taste. Upon notifying the Manchester Water Company, water samples were taken and preliminary analysis disclosed that the contaminants found were not the typical contaminants associated with fire line disturbances. Investigating teams suspected that either the nearby fire could have siphoned contaminants from adjacent buildings into the water mains, or the contamination could have been caused by a plumbing deficiency occurring within the seven story building itself.

Water ph levels of the building water indicated that an injection of chemicals had probably taken place within the seven-story building. Tracing of the water lines within the building pinpointed a 10,000 gallon hot-water storage tank that was used for heat storage in the solar heating system. It did not have any backflow protection on the make-up

supply line! As the storage tank pressure increased above the supply pressure, as a result of thermal expansion, the potential for backpressure backflow was present. Normally, this would not occur because a boost pump in the supply line would keep the supply pressure to the storage tank always greater than the highest tank pressure. The addition of rust inhibiting chemicals to this tank greatly increased the degree of hazard of the liquid. Unfortunately, at the same time that the fire took place, the pressure in the water mains was reduced to a dangerously low pressure and the low pressure cutoff switches simultaneously shut off the storage tank booster pumps. This combination allowed the boiler water, together with its chemical contaminants, the opportunity to enter the potable water supply within the building. When normal pressure was reestablished in the water mains, the booster pumps kicked in, and the contaminated water was delivered throughout the building.

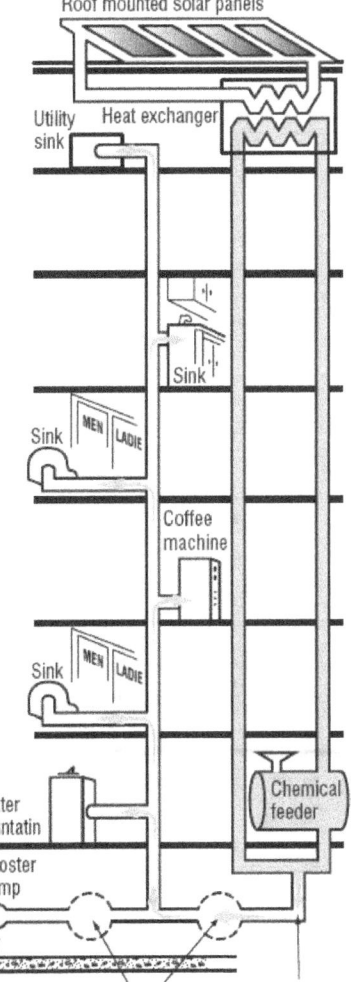

Roof mounted solar panels

Utility sink   Heat exchanger

Sink

Sink   MEN | LADIE

Coffee machine

Sink   MEN | LADIE

Chemical feeder

Water fountatin

Booster pump

Meter

Water main

Recommended installation of backflow preventers

Backpressure backflow

Dialysis Machine Contamination

Ethylene glycol, an anti-freeze additive to air conditioning cooling tower water, inadvertently entered the potable water supply system in a medical center in Illinois in September, 1982, and two of six dialysis patients succumbed as a direct or indirect result of the contamination.

The glycol was added to the air conditioning water, and the glycol/water mix was stored in a holding tank that was an integral part of the medical center's air conditioning cooling system. Pressurized make-up water to the holding tank was supplied by a medical center potable supply line and fed through a manually operated control valve. With this valve open, or partially open, potable make-up water flowed slowly into the glycol/water mixture in the holding tank until it filled to the point where the pressure in the closed tank equaled the pressure in the potable water supply feed line. As long as the potable feed line pressure was at least equal to, or greater than, the holding tank pressure, no backflow could occur. The stage was set for disaster, however.

It was theorized that someone in the medical center flushed a toilet or turned on a faucet, which in turn dropped the pressure in the potable supply line to the air conditioning holding tank. Since the manually operated fill valve was partially open, this allowed the glycol/water mixture to enter the medical center potable pipelines and flow into the dialysis equipment. The dialysis filtration system takes out trace chemicals such as those used in the city water treatment plant, but the system could not handle the heavy load of chemicals that it was suddenly subjected to.

The effect upon the dialysis patients was dramatic: patients became drowsy, confused and fell unconscious, and were promptly removed to intensive care where blood samples were taken. The blood samples revealed a build-up of acid and the medical director stated that, "Something has happened in dialysis." Dialysis was repeated on the patients a second and third time.

Tests of the water supply to the filtration system quickly determined the presence of "an undesirable chemical in the water purification system." The partially open fill valve was then found that it had permitted the glycol water mix to drain from the air conditioning holding tank into the medical center's potable supply lines and then into the dialysis filtration system equipment.

Creosote in the Water Mains

Creosote entered the water distribution system of a southeastern county water authority in Georgia, in November, 1984, as a result of cross-connection between a ¾-inch hose that was being used as a priming line between a fire service connection and the suction side of a creosote pump. The hose continually supplied water to the pump to ensure the pump was primed at all times. However, while repairs were being made to a private fire hydrant, the creosote back-siphoned into the water mains and contaminated a section of the water distribution system.

Detailed investigation of the cause of the incident disclosed that the wood preservative company, as part of their operation, pumped creosote from collective pits to other parts of their operation. The creosote pump would automatically shut off when the creosote in the pit was lowered to a predetermined level. After the creosote returned to a higher level, the pump would restart. This pump would lose its prime quite often prior to the pit refilling, and to prevent the loss of prime, the wood preservative company would connect a hose from a ¾-inch hose bibb, located on the fire service line, to the suction side of the pump. The hose bibb remained open at all times in an effort to continuously keep the pump primed.

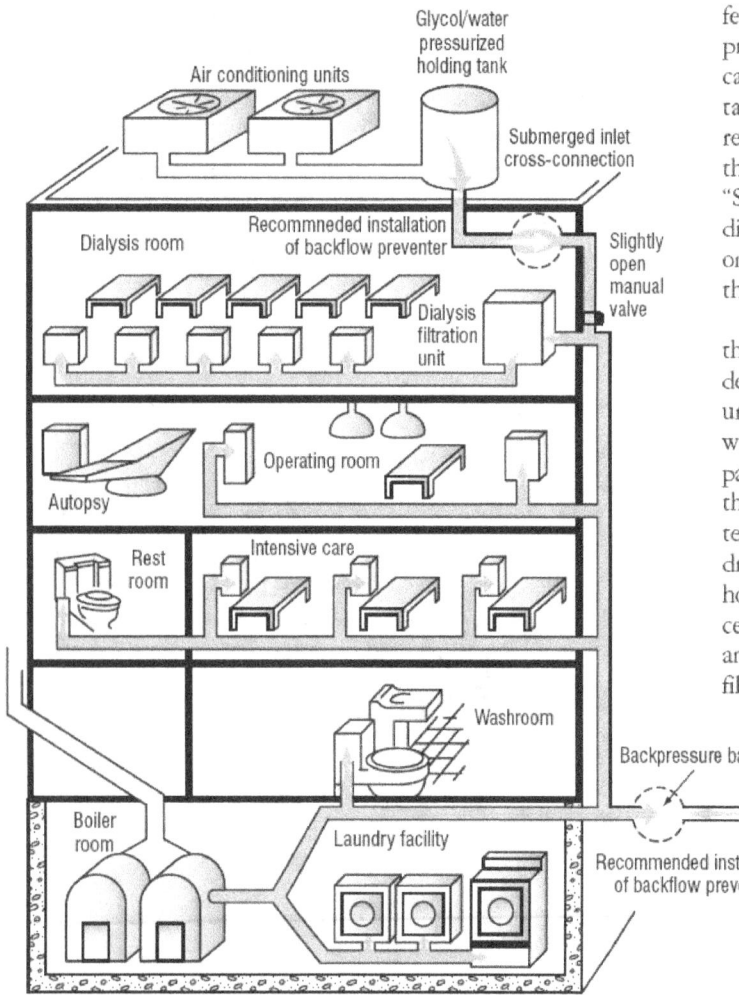

![Street main diagram showing creosote contamination flow through houses]

Street main

Creosote pump

Process water

Private shut-off

Recommended installation of backflow preventers

Recommended installation of backflow preventers

Street main

Creosote contaminated flow

Kool-Aid Laced With Chlordane

In August, 1978, a professional exterminator was treating a church located in a small town in South Carolina, for termite and pest control. The highly toxic insecticide chlordane was being mixed with water in small buckets, and garden hoses were left submerged in the buckets while the mixing was being accomplished. At the same time, water department personnel came by to disconnect the parsonage's water line from the church to install a separate water meter for the parsonage. In the process, the water was shut off in the area of the church building. Since the church was located on a steep hill, and as the remaining water in the lines was used by residents in the area, the church was among the first places to experience a negative pressure.

The chlordane was quickly siphoned into the water lines within the church and became mixed with the Kool-Aid being prepared by women for the vacation bible school. Approximately a dozen children and three adults experienced dizziness and nausea. Fortunately, none required hospitalization or medical attention.

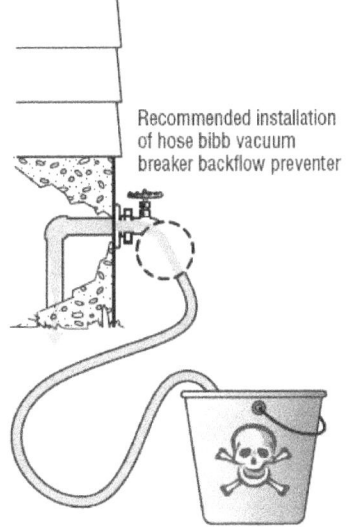

Recommended installation of hose bibb vacuum breaker backflow preventer

Repairs were necessary to one of the private fire hydrants on the wood preservative company property, necessitating the shutting down of one of two service lines and removal of the damaged fire hydrant for repair. Since the hydrant was at a significantly lower level than the creosote pit, the creosote back-siphoned through a ¾-inch pump priming hose connecting the creosote pit to the fire service line.

After the repairs were made to the hydrant, and the water service restored, the creosote, now in the fire lines, was forced into the main water distribution system.

Chapter Three

Theory of Backflow and Backsiphonage

$$P_{absolute} = P_{gage} + 14.7 psi$$
or
$$P_{gage} = P_{absolute} - 14.7 psi$$

A cross-connection[1] is the link or channel connecting a source of pollution with a potable water supply. The polluting substance, in most cases a liquid, tends to enter the potable supply if the net force acting upon the liquid acts in the direction of the potable supply. Two factors are therefore essential for backflow. First, there must be a link between the two systems. Second, the resultant force must be toward the potable supply.

An understanding of the principles of backflow and backsiphonage requires an understanding of the terms frequently used in their discussion. *Force,* unless completely resisted, will produce motion. Weight is a type of force resulting from the earth's gravitational attraction. Pressure (P) is a force-per-unit area, such as pounds per square inch (psi). *Atmospheric pressure* is the pressure exerted by the weight of the atmosphere above the earth.

Pressure may be referred to using an absolute scale, pounds per square inch absolute (psia), or gage scale, pounds per square inch gage (psig). Absolute pressure and gage pressure are related. Absolute pressure is equal to the gage pressure plus the atmospheric pressure. At sea level the atmospheric pressure is 14.7 psia. Thus,

In essence then, absolute pressure is the total pressure. Gage pressure is simply the pressure read on a gage. If there is no pressure on the gage other than atmospheric, the gage would read zero. Then the absolute pressure would be equal to 14.7 psi which is the atmospheric pressure.

The term *vacuum* indicates that the absolute pressure is less than the atmospheric pressure and that the gage pressure is negative. A complete or total vacuum would mean a pressure of 0 psia or -14.7 psig. Since it is impossible to produce a total vacuum, the term vacuum, as used in the text, will mean all degrees of partial vacuum. In a partial vacuum, the pressure would range from slightly less than 14.7 psia (0 psig) to slightly greater than 0 psia (-14.7 psig).

Backsiphonage[1] results in fluid flow in an undesirable or reverse direction. It is caused by atmospheric pressure exerted on a pollutant liquid forcing it toward a potable water supply system that is under a vacuum. Backflow, although literally meaning any type of reversed flow, refers to the flow produced by the differential pressure existing between two systems both of which are at pressures greater than atmospheric.

Water Pressure

For an understanding of the nature of pressure and its relationship to water depth, consider the pressure exerted on the base of a cubic foot of water at sea level. (See Fig. 1) The average weight of a cubic foot of water is 62.4 pounds per square foot gage. The base may be subdivided into 144-square inches with each subdivision being subjected to a pressure of 0.433 psig.

Suppose another cubic foot of water were placed directly on top of the first (See Fig. 2). The pressure on the top surface of the first cube which was originally atmospheric, or 0 psig, would now be 0.433 psig as a result of the superimposed cubic foot of water. The pressure of the base of the first cube would also be increased by the same amount of 0.866 psig, or two times the original pressure.

FIGURE 1.
Pressure exerted by 1 foot of water at sea level.

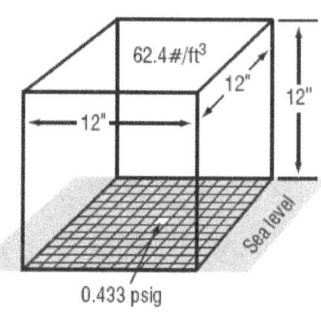

[1]See formal definition in the glossary of the appendix

If this process were repeated with a third cubic foot of water, the pressures at the base of each cube would be 1,299 psig, 0.866 psig, and 0.433 psig, respectively. It is evident that pressure varies with depth below a free water surface; in general each foot of elevation change, within a liquid, changes the pressure by an amount equal to the weight-per-unit area of 1 foot of the liquid. The rate of increase for water is 0.433 psi per foot of depth.

Frequently water pressure is referred to using the terms "pressure head" or just "head," and is expressed in units of feet of water. One foot of head would be equivalent to the pressure produced at the base of a column of water 1 foot in depth. One foot of head or 1 foot of water is equal to 0.433 psig. One hundred feet of head is equal to 43.3 psig.

FIGURE 2.
Pressure exerted by 2 feet of water at sea level.

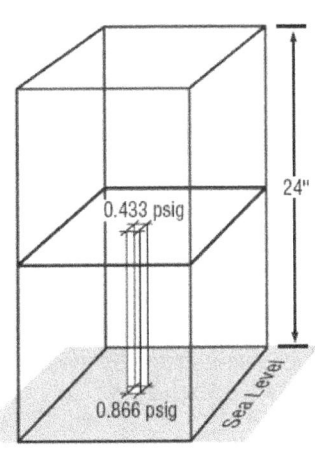

1See formal definition in the glossary of the appendix

Siphon Theory

Figure 3 depicts the atmospheric pressure on a water surface at sea level. An open tube is inserted vertically into the water; atmospheric pressure, which is 14.7 psia, acts equally on the surface of the water within the tube and on the outside of the tube.

FIGURE 3.
Pressure on the free surface of a liquid at sea level.

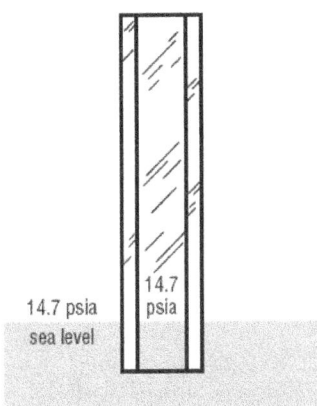

If, as shown in Figure 4, the tube is slightly capped and a vacuum pump is used to evacuate all the air from the sealed tube, a vacuum with a pressure of 0 psia is created within the tube. Because the pressure at any point in a static fluid is dependent upon the height of that point above a reference line, such as sea level, it follows that the pressure within the tube at sea level must still be 14.7 psia. This is equivalent to the pressure at the base of a column of water 33.9 feet high and with the column open at the base, water would rise to fill the column to a depth of 33.9 feet. In other words, the weight of the atmosphere at sea

level exactly balances the weight of a column of water 33.9 feet in height. The absolute pressure within the column of water in Figure 4 at a height of 11.5 feet is equal to 9.7 psia. This is a partial vacuum with an equivalent gage pressure of -5.0 psig.

As a practical example, assume the water pressure at a closed faucet on the top of a 100-foot high building to be 20 psig; the pressure on the ground floor would then be 63.3 psig. If the pressure at the ground were to drop suddenly due to a heavy fire demand in the area to 33.3 psig, the pressure at the top would be reduced to -10 psig. If the building water system were airtight, the water would remain at the level of the faucet

FIGURE 4.
Effect of evacuating air from a column.

because of the partial vacuum created by the drop in pressure. If the faucet were opened, however, the vacuum would be broken and the water level would drop to a height of 77 feet above the ground. Thus, the atmosphere was supporting a column of water 23 feet high.

Figure 5 is a diagram of an inverted U-tube that has been filled with water and placed in two open containers at sea level.

If the open containers are placed so that the liquid levels in each container are at the same height, a static state will exist; and the pressure at any specified level in either leg of the U-tube will be the same.

The equilibrium condition is altered by raising one of the containers so that the liquid level in one container is 5 feet

FIGURE 5.
Pressure relationships in a continuous fluid system at the same elevation.

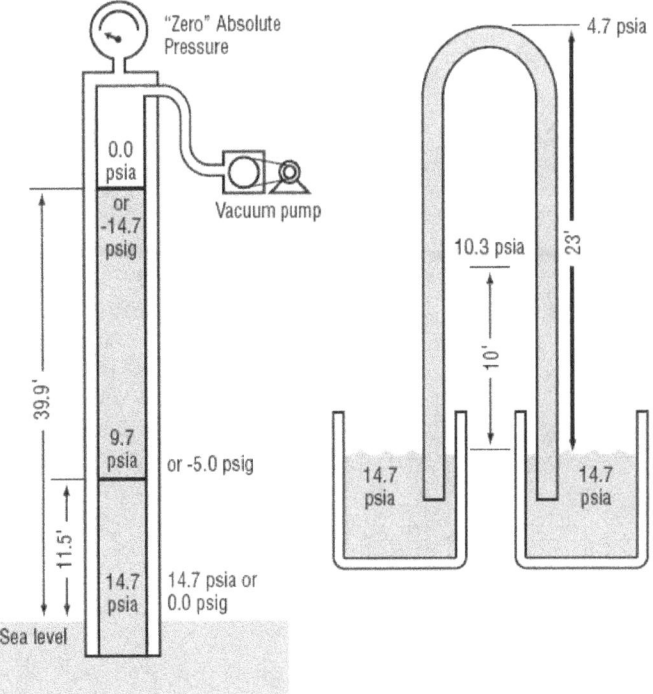

above the level of the other. (See Fig. 6.) Since both containers are open to the atmosphere, the pressure on the liquid surfaces in each container will remain at 14.7 psia.

If it is assumed that a static state exists, momentarily, within the system shown in Figure 6, the pressure in the left tube at any height above the free surface in the left container can be calculated. The pressure at the corresponding level in the right tube above the free surface in the right container may also be calculated.

As shown in Figure 6, the pressure at all levels in the left tube would be less than at corresponding levels in the right tube. In this case, a static condition cannot exist because fluid will flow from the higher pressure to the lower pressure; the flow would be from the right tank to the left tank. This arrangement will be recognized as a siphon. The crest of a siphon cannot be higher than 33.9 feet above the upper liquid

FIGURE 6.
Pressure relationships in a continuous fluid system at different elevations.

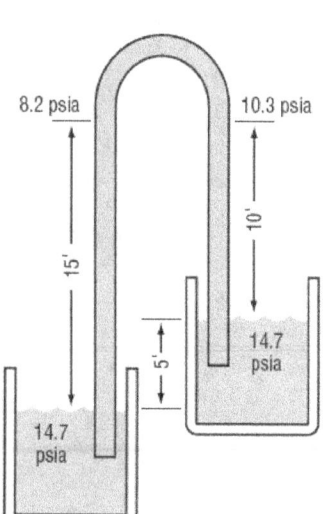

level, since atmosphere cannot support a column of water greater in height than 33.9 feet.

Figure 7 illustrates how this siphon principle can be hazardous in a plumbing system. If the supply valve is closed, the pressure in the line supplying the faucet is less than the pressure in the supply line to the bathtub. Flow will occur, therefore, through siphonage, from the bathtub to the open faucet.

FIGURE 7.
Backsiphonage in a plumbing system.

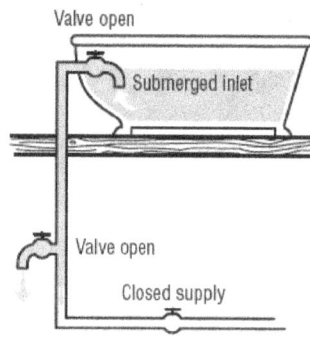

The siphon actions cited have been produced by reduced pressures resulting from a difference in the water levels at two separated points within a continuous fluid system.

Reduced pressure may also be created within a fluid system as a result of fluid motion. One of the basic principles of fluid mechanics is the principle of conservation of energy. Based upon this principle, it may be

shown that as a fluid accelerates, as shown in Figure 8, the pressure is reduced. As water flows through a constriction such as a converging section of pipe, the velocity of the water increases; as a result, the pressure is reduced. Under such conditions, negative pressures may be developed in a pipe. The simple aspirator is based upon this principle. If this point of reduced pressure is linked to a source of pollution, backsiphonage of the pollutant can occur.

FIGURE 8.
Negative pressure created by constricted flow.

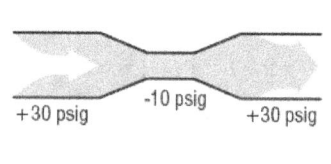

One of the common occurrences of dynamically reduced pipe pressures is found on the suction side of a pump. In many cases similar to the one illustrated in Figure 9, the line supplying the booster pump is undersized or does not have sufficient pressure to deliver water at the rate at which the pump normally operates. The rate of flow in the pipe may be increased by a further reduction in pressure at the pump intake. This often results in the creation of negative pressure at the pump intake. This often results in the creation of negative pressure. This negative pressure may become low enough in some cases to cause vaporization of the water in the line. Actually, in the illustration shown,

FIGURE 9.
Dynamically reduced pipe pressures.

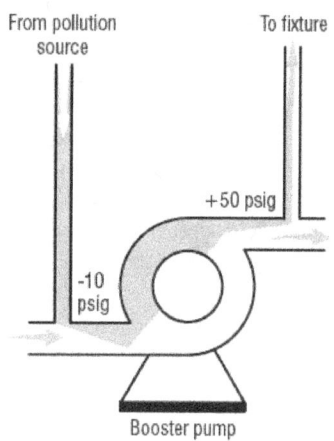

flow from the source of pollution would occur when pressure on the suction side of the pump is less than pressure of the pollution source; but this is *backflow,* which will be discussed below.

The preceding discussion has described some of the means by which negative pressures may be created and which frequently occur to produce backsiphonage. In addition to the negative pressure or reversed force necessary to cause backsiphonage and backflow, there must also be the cross-connection or connecting link between the potable water supply and the source of pollution. Two basic types of connections may be created in piping systems. These are the solid pipe with valved connection and the *submerged inlet.*

Figures 10 and 11 illustrate solid connections. This type of connection is often installed where it is necessary to supply an auxiliary piping system from the potable source. It is a direct connection of one pipe to another pipe or receptacle.

Solid pipe connections are often made to continuous or intermittent waste lines where it is assumed that the flow will be in one direction only. An example of this would be used cooling water from a water jacket or condenser as shown in Figure 11. This type of connection is usually detectable but creating a concern on the part of the installer about the possibility of reversed flow is often more difficult. Upon questioning, however, many installers will agree that the solid connection was made because the sewer is occasionally subjected to backpressure.

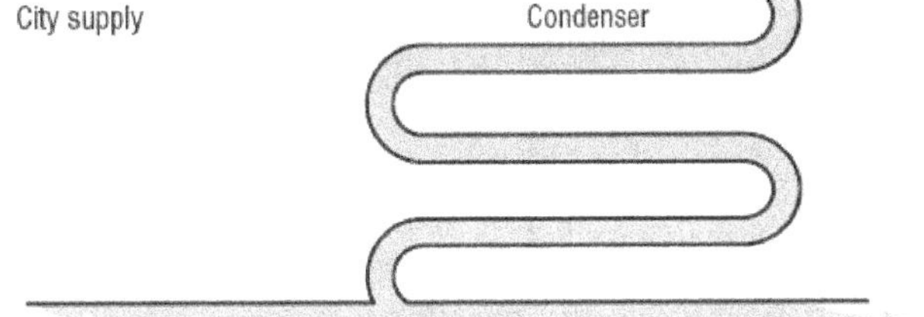

Submerged inlets are found on many common plumbing fixtures and are sometimes necessary features of the fixtures if they are to function properly. Examples of this type of design are siphon-jet urinals or water closets, flushing rim slop sinks, and dental cuspidors. Oldstyle bathtubs and lavatories had supply inlets below the flood level rims, but modern sanitary design has minimized or eliminated this hazard in new fixtures. Chemical and industrial process vats sometimes have submerged inlets where the water pressure is used as an aid in diffusion, dispersion and agitation of the vat contents. Even though the supply pipe may come from the floor above the vat, backsiphonage can occur as it has been shown that the siphon action can raise a liquid such as water almost 34 feet. Some submerged inlets

difficult to control are those which are not apparent until a significant change in water level occurs or where a supply may be conveniently extended below the liquid surface by means of a hose or auxiliary piping. A submerged inlet may be created in numerous ways, and its detection in some of these subtle forms may be difficult.

The illustrations included in part B of the appendix are intended to describe typical examples of backsiphonage, showing in each case the nature of the link or cross-connection, and the cause of the negative pressure.

Backflow

Backflow[1], as described in this manual, refers to reversed flow due to backpressure other than siphonic action. Any interconnected fluid systems in which the pressure of one exceeds the pressure of the other may have flow from one to the other as a result of the pressure differential. The flow will occur from the zone of higher pressure to the zone of lower pressure. This type of backflow is of concern in buildings where two or more piping systems are maintained. The potable water supply is usually under pressure directly from the city water main. Occasionally, a booster pump is used. The auxiliary system is often pressurized by a centrifical pump, although backpressure may be caused by gas or steam pressure from a boiler. A

reversal in differential pressure may occur when pressure in the potable system drops, for some reason, to a pressure lower than that in the system to which the potable water is connected.

The most positive method of avoiding this type of backflow is the total or complete separation of the two systems. Other methods used involve the installation of mechanical devices. All methods require routine inspection and maintenance.

Dual piping systems are often installed for extra protection in the event of an emergency or possible mechanical failure of one of the systems. Fire protection systems are an example. Another example is the use of dual water connections to boilers. These installations are sometimes interconnected, thus creating a health hazard.

The illustrations in part C of the appendix depict installations where backflow under pressure can occur, describing the cross-connection and the cause of the reversed flow.

FIGURE 10.
Valved connections between potable water and nonpotable fluid.

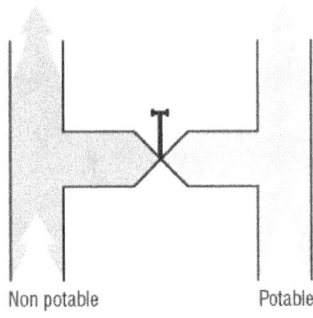

Non potable   Potable

FIGURE 11
Valved connection between potable water and sanitary sewer.

City supply   Condenser

Sanitary sewer

[1]See formal definition in the glossary of the appendix

Chapter Four

Methods and Devices for the Prevention of Backflow and Back-Siphonage

A wide choice of devices exists that can be used to prevent backsiphonage and backpressure from adding contaminated fluids or gases into a potable water supply system. Generally, the selection of the proper device to use is based upon the degree of hazard posed by the cross-connection. Additional considerations are based upon piping size, location, and the potential need to periodically test the devices to insure proper operation.

There are six basic types of devices that can be used to correct cross-connections: air gaps, barometric loops, vacuum breakers—both atmospheric and pressure type, double check with intermediate atmospheric vent, double check valve assemblies, and reduced pressure principle devices. In general, all manufacturers of these devices, with the exception of the barometric loop, produce them to one or more of three basic standards, thus insuring the public that dependable devices are being utilized and marketed. The major standards in the industry are: American Society of Sanitary Engineers ASSE), American Water Works Association (AWWA), and the University of California Foundation for Cross-Connection Control and Hydraulic Research.

Air Gap

Air gaps are non-mechanical backflow preventers that are very effective devices to be used where either backsiphonage or backpressure conditions may exist. Their use is as old as piping and plumbing itself, but only relatively recently have standards been issued that standardize their design. In general, the air gap must be twice the supply pipe diameter but never less than one inch. See Figure 12.

FIGURE 12.
Air gap.

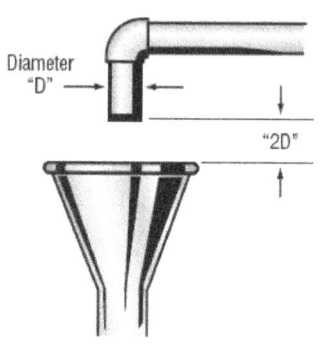

An air gap, although an extremely effective backflow preventer when used to prevent backsiphonage and backpressure conditions, does interrupt the piping flow with corresponding loss of pressure for subsequent use. Consequently, air gaps are primarily used at end of the line service where reservoirs or storage tanks are desired. When contemplating the use of an air gap, some other considerations are:

(1) In a continuous piping system, each air gap requires the added expense of reservoirs and secondary pumping systems.

(2) The air gap may be easily defeated in the event that the "2D" requirement was purposely or inadvertently compromised. Excessive splash may be encountered in the event that higher than anticipated pressures or flows occur. The splash may be a cosmetic or true potential hazard—the simple solution being to reduce the "2D" dimension by thrusting the supply pipe into the receiving funnel. By so doing, the air gap is defeated.

(3) At an air gap, we expose the water to the surrounding air with its inherent bacteria, dust particles, and other airborne pollutants or contaminants. In addition, the aspiration effect of the flowing water can drag down surrounding pollutants into the reservoir or holding tank.

(4) Free chlorine can come out of treated water as a result of the air gap and the resulting splash and churning effect as the water enters the holding tanks. This reduces the ability of the water to withstand bacteria contamination during long term storage.

(5) For the above reasons, air gaps must be inspected as frequently as mechanical backflow preventers. They are not exempt from an in-depth cross-connection control program requiring periodic inspection of all backflow devices.

Air gaps may be fabricated from commercially available plumbing components or purchased as separate units and integrated into plumbing and piping systems. An example of the use of an air gap is shown in Figure 13.

FIGURE 13.
Air gap in a piping system.

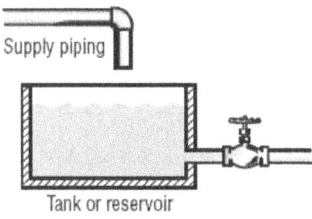

Supply piping

Tank or reservoir

Barometric Loop

The barometric loop consists of a continuous section of supply piping that abruptly rises to a height of approximately 35 feet and then returns back down to the originating level. It is a loop in the piping system that effectively protects against backsiphonage. It may not be used to protect against backpressure.

Its operation, in the protection against backsiphonage, is based upon the principle that a water column, at sea level pressure, will not rise above 33.9 feet (Ref. Chapter 3, Fig. 4 Page 13).

In general, barometric loops are locally fabricated, and are 35 feet high.

FIGURE 14.
Barometric loop.

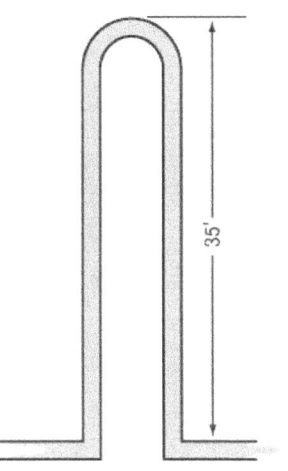

35'

Atmospheric Vacuum Breaker

These devices are among the simplest and least expensive mechanical types of backflow preventers and, when installed properly, can provide excellent protection against back-siphonage. They must not be utilized to protect against backpressure conditions. Construction consists usually of a polyethylene float which is free to travel on a shaft and seal in the uppermost position against atmosphere with an elastomeric disc. Water flow lifts the float, which then causes the disc to seal. Water pressure keeps the float in the upward sealed position. Termination of the water supply will cause the disc to drop down venting the unit to atmosphere and thereby opening downstream piping to atmospheric pressure, thus preventing backsiphonage. Figure 15 shows a typical atmospheric breaker.

In general, these devices are available in ½-inch through 3-inch size and must be installed vertically, must not have shutoffs downstream, and must be installed at least 6-inches higher than the final outlet. They cannot be tested once they are installed in the plumbing system, but are, for the most part, dependable, trouble-free devices for backsiphonage protection.

FIGURE 15.
Atmospheric vacuum breaker.

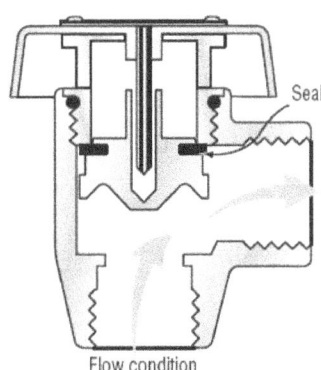

Seal

Flow condition

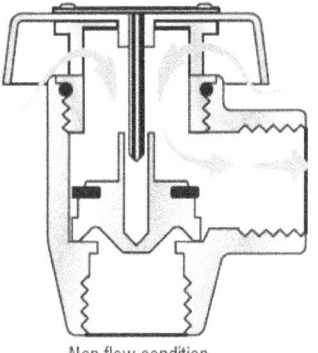

Non flow condition

Figure 16 shows the generally accepted installation requirements—note that no shutoff valve is downstream of the device that would otherwise keep the atmospheric vacuum breaker under constant pressure.

Figure 17 shows a typical installation of an atmospheric vacuum breaker in a plumbing supply system.

FIGURE 16.
Atmospheric vacuum breaker typical installation.

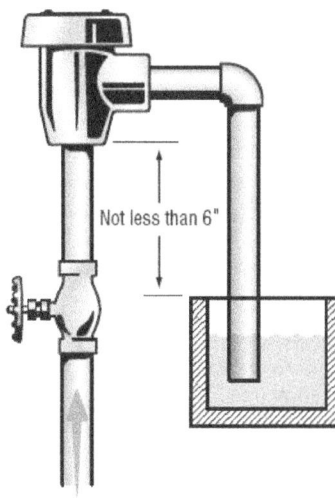

Not less than 6"

FIGURE 17.
Atmospheric vacuum breaker in plumbing supply system.

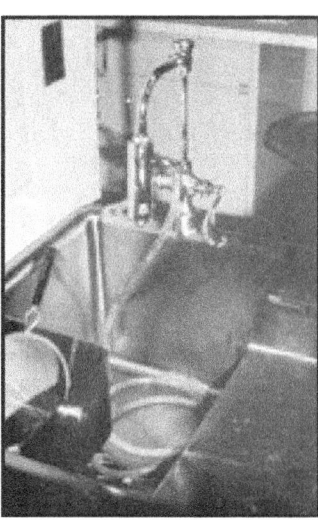

Hose Bibb Vacuum Breakers

These small devices are a specialized application of the atmospheric vacuum breaker. They are generally attached to sill cocks and in turn are connected to hose supplied outlets such as garden hoses, slop sink hoses, spray outlets, etc. They consist of a spring loaded check valve that seals against an atmospheric outlet when water supply pressure is turned on. Typical construction is shown in Figure 18.

When the water supply is turned off, the device vents to atmosphere, thus protecting against backsiphonage conditions. They should not be used as backpressure devices. Manual drain options are available, together with tamper-proof versions. A typical installation is shown in Figure 19.

FIGURE 19.
Typical installation of hose bibb vacuum breaker.

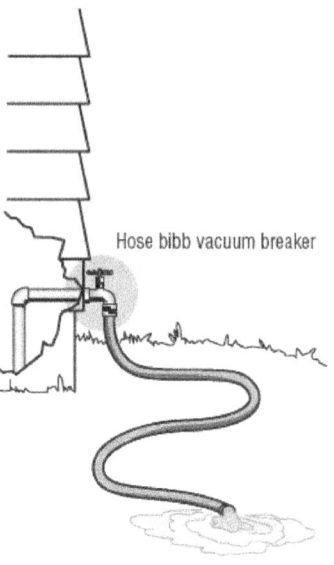

Hose bibb vacuum breaker

Pressure Vacuum Breakers

This device is an outgrowth of the atmospheric vacuum breaker and evolved in response to a need to have an atmospheric vacuum breaker that could be utilized under constant pressure and that could be tested in line. A spring on top of the disc and float assembly, two added gate valves, test cocks, and an additional first check, provided the answer to achieve this device. See Figure 20.

These units are available in the general configurations as shown in Figure 20 in sizes ½-inch through 10-inch and have broad usage in the agriculture and irrigation market. Typical agricultural and industrial applications are shown in Figure 21.

Again, these devices may be used under constant pressure but do not protect against backpressure conditions. As a result, installation must be at least 6- to 12-inches higher than the existing outlet.

A spill resistant pressure vacuum breaker (SVB) is available that is a modification to the standard pressure vacuum breaker but specifically designed to minimize water spillage. Installation and hydraulic requirements are similar to the standard pressure vacuum breaker and the devices are recommended for internal use.

FIGURE 20.
Pressure vacuum breaker

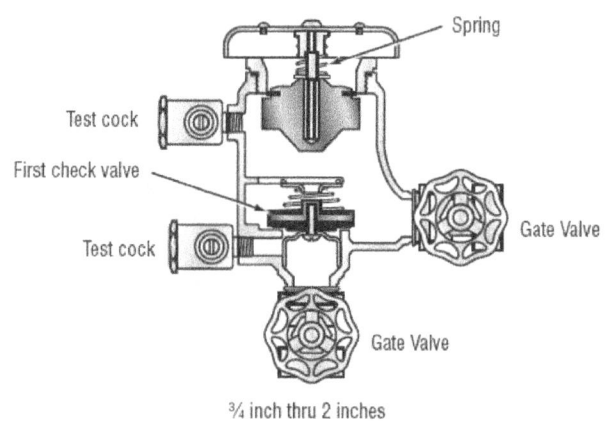

Spring

Test cock

First check valve

Test cock

Gate Valve

Gate Valve

¾ inch thru 2 inches

2½ inches thru 10 inches

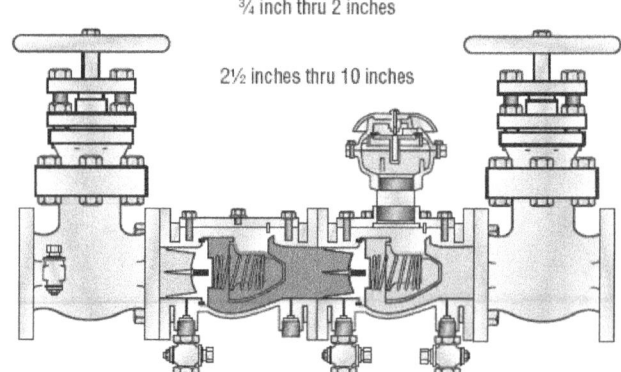

FIGURE 18.
Hose bibb vacuum breaker.

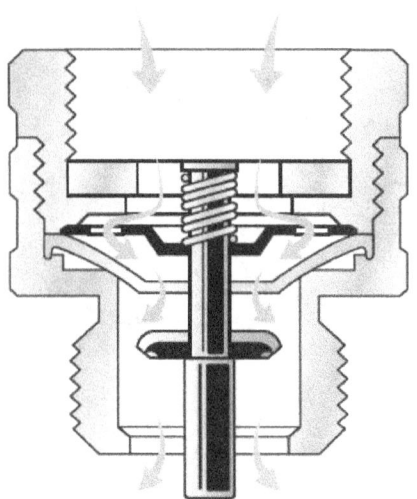

Double Check with Intermediate Atmospheric Vent

The need to provide a compact device in ½-inch and ¾-inch pipe sizes that protects against moderate hazards, is capable of being used under constant pressure and that protects against backpressure, resulted in this unique backflow preventer. Construction is basically a double check valve having an atmospheric vent located between the two checks (See Figure 22).

Line pressure keeps the vent closed, but zero supply pressure or backsiphonage will open the inner chamber to atmosphere. With this device, extra protection is obtained through the atmospheric vent capability. Figure 23 shows a typical use of the device on a residential boiler supply line.

FIGURE 21.
Typical agricultural and industrial application of pressure vacuum breaker.

FIGURE 22.
Double check valve with atmospheric vent.

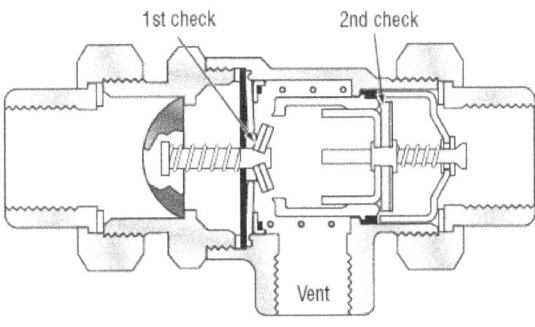

1st check   2nd check

Vent

FIGURE 23.
Typical residential use of double check with atmospheric vent.

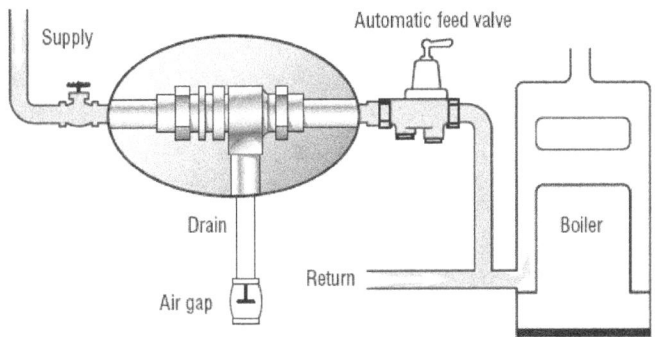

Supply

Automatic feed valve

Drain

Boiler

Air gap

Return

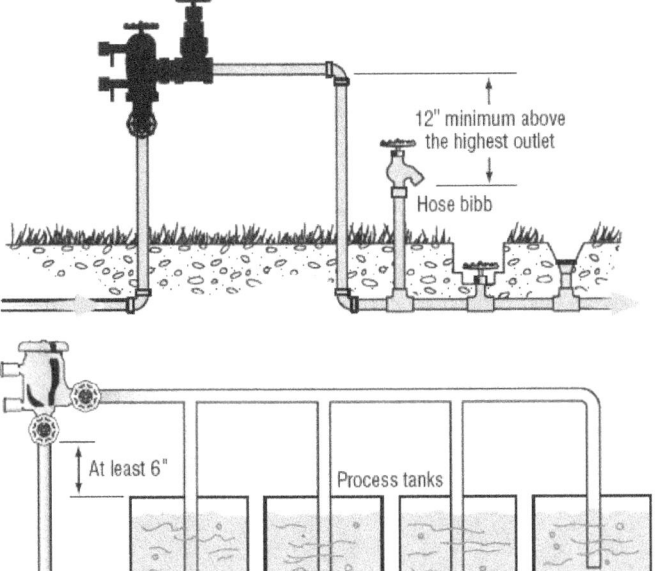

12" minimum above the highest outlet

Hose bibb

At least 6"

Process tanks

Double Check Valve

A double check valve is essentially two single check valves coupled within one body and furnished with test cocks and two tightly closing gate valves (See Figure 24).

The test capability feature gives this device a big advantage over the use of two independent check valves in that it can be readily tested to determine if either or both check valves are inoperative or fouled by debris. Each check is spring loaded closed and requires approximately a pound of pressure to open.

This spring loading provides the ability to "bite" through small debris and still seal—a protection feature not prevalent in unloaded swing check valves. Figure 24 shows a cross section of double check valve complete with test cocks. Double checks are commonly used to protect against low to medium hazard installations such as food processing steam kettles and apartment projects. They may be used under continuous pressure and protect against both backsiphonage and backpressure conditions.

FIGURE 24.
Double check valve.

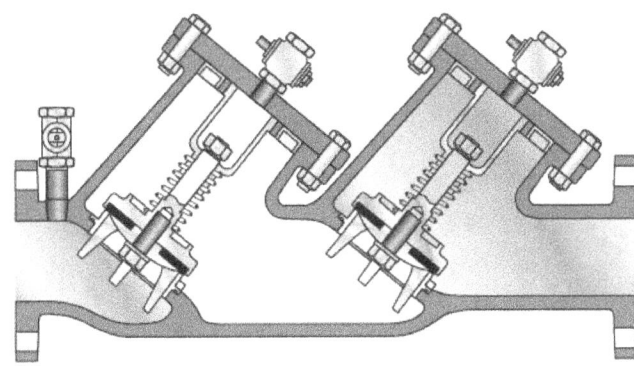

Double Check Detector Check

This device is an outgrowth of the double check valve and is primarily utilized in fire line installations. Its purpose is to protect the potable supply line from possible contamination or pollution from fire line chemical additives, booster pump fire line backpressure, stagnant "black water" that sits in fire lines over extended periods of time, the addition of "raw" water through outside fire pumper connections (Siamese outlets), and the detection of any water movement in the fire line water due to fire line leakage or deliberate water theft. It consists of two, spring loaded check valves, a bypass assembly with water meter and double check valve, and two tightly closing gate valves. See Figure 25. The addition of test cocks makes the device testable

FIGURE 25.
Double check detector check.

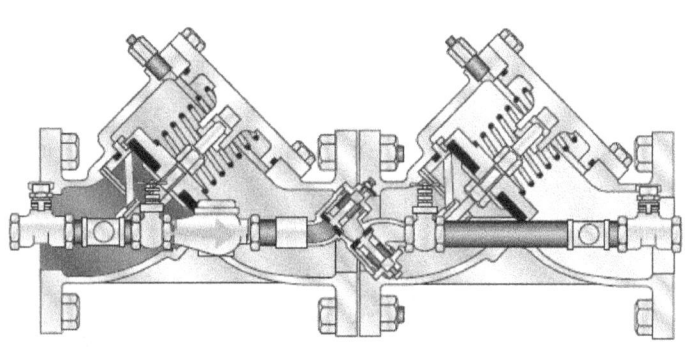

to insure proper operation of both the primary checks and the bypass check valve. In the event of very low fire line water usage, (theft of water) the low pressure drop inherent in the bypass system permits the low flow of water to be metered through the bypass system. In a high flow demand, associated with deluge fire capability, the main check valves open, permitting high volume, low restricted flow, through the two large spring loaded check valves.

Residential Dual Check

The need to furnish reliable and inexpensive backsiphonage and backpressure protection for individual residences resulted in the debut of the residential dual check. Protection of the main potable supply from household hazards such as home photograph chemicals, toxic insect and garden sprays, termite control pesticides used by exterminators, etc., reinforced, a true need for such a device. Figure 26 shows a cutaway of the device.

FIGURE 26.
Residential dual check.

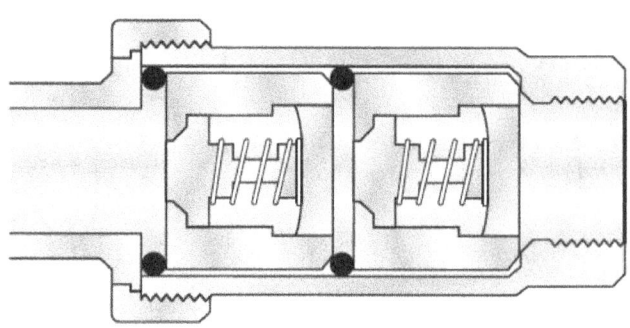

It is sized for ½-, ¾-, and 1-inch service lines and is installed immediately downstream of the water meter. The use of plastic check modules and elimination of test cocks and gate valves keeps the cost reasonable while providing good, dependable protection. Typical installations are shown in Figures 27 and 28.

FIGURE 27.
Residential Installation.

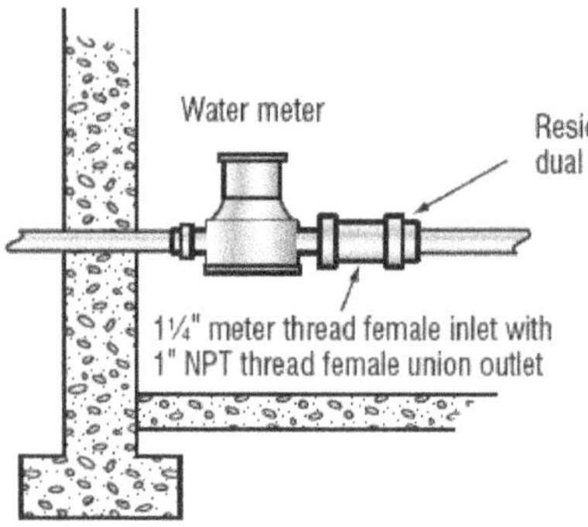

Water meter

1¼" meter thread female inlet with 1" NPT thread female union outlet

FIGURE 28.
Copper horn.

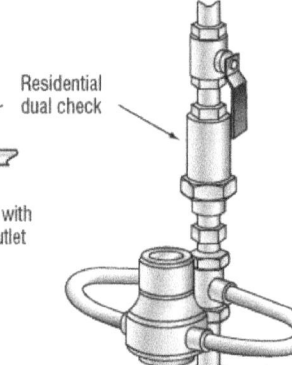

Residential dual check

Water meter

Reduced Pressure Principle Backflow Preventer

Maximum protection is achieved against backsiphonage and backpressure conditions utilizing reduced pressure principle backflow preventers. These devices are essentially modified double check valves with an atmospheric vent capability placed between the two checks and designed such that this "zone" between the two checks is always kept at least two pounds less than the supply pressure. With this design criteria, the reduced pressure principle backflow preventer can provide protection against backsiphonage and backpressure when both the first and second checks become fouled. They can be used under constant pressure and at high hazard installations. They are furnished with test cocks and gate valves to enable testing and are available in sizes ¾-inch through 10 inch.

Figure 29A shows typical devices representative of ¾-inch through 2-inch size and Figure 29B shows typical devices representative of 2½-inch through 10-inch sizes.

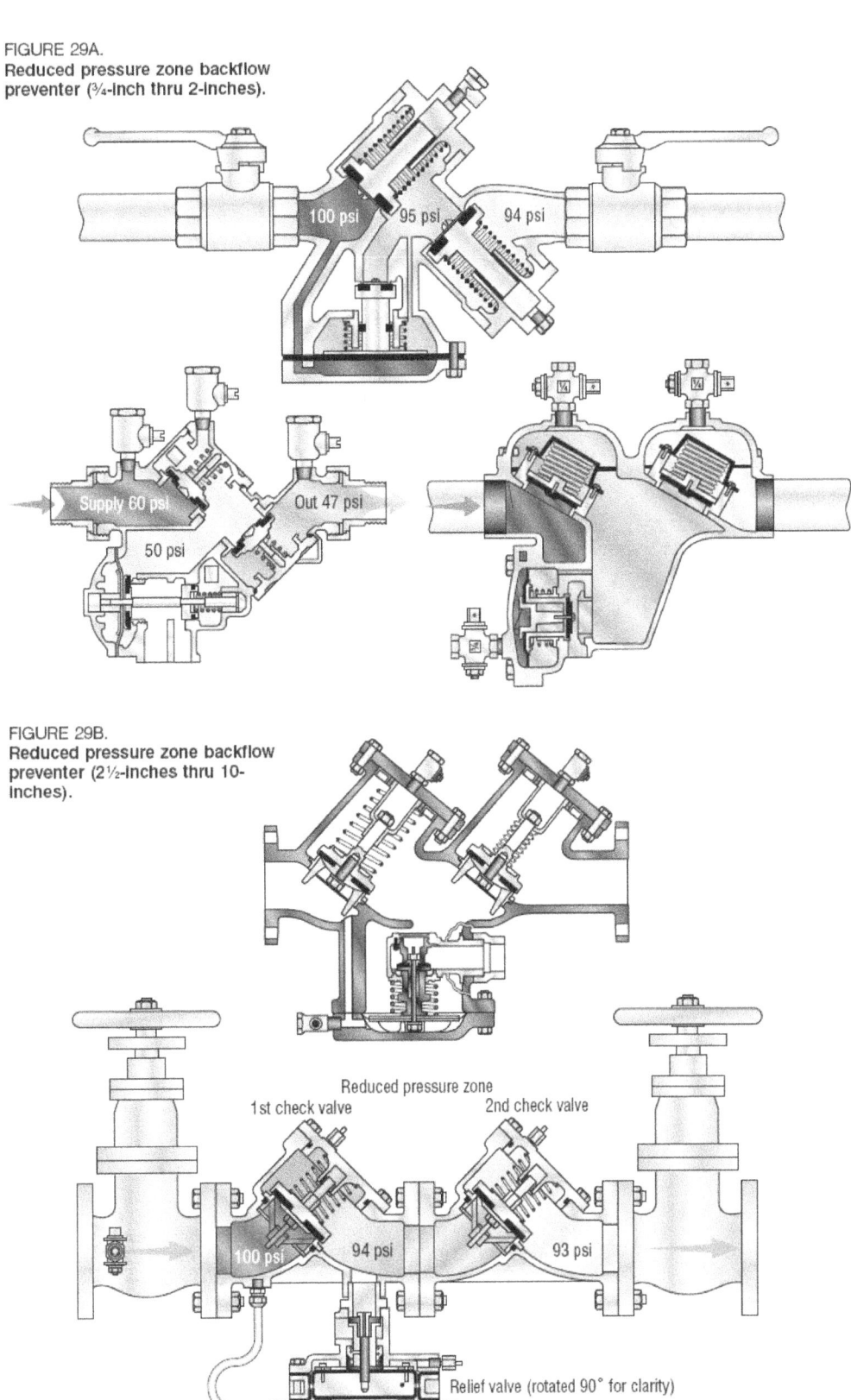

FIGURE 29A.
Reduced pressure zone backflow preventer (¾-inch thru 2-inches).

FIGURE 29B.
Reduced pressure zone backflow preventer (2½-inches thru 10-inches).

The principles of operation of a reduced pressure principle backflow preventer are as follows:

Flow from the left enters the central chamber against the pressure exerted by the loaded check valve 1. The supply pressure is reduced thereupon by a predetermined amount. The pressure in the central chamber is maintained lower than the incoming supply pressure through the operation of the relief valve 3, which discharges to the atmosphere whenever the central chamber pressure approaches within a few pounds of the inlet pressure. Check valve 2 is lightly loaded to open with a pressure drop of 1 psi in the direction of flow and is independent of the pressure required to open the relief valve. In the event that the pressure increases downstream from the device, tending to reverse the direction of flow, check valve 2 closes, preventing backflow. Because all valves may leak as a result of wear or obstruction, the protection provided by the check valves is not considered sufficient. If some obstruction prevents check valve 2 from closing tightly, the leakage back into the central chamber would increase the pressure in this zone, the relief valve would open, and flow would be discharged to the atmosphere.

When the supply pressure drops to the minimum differential required to operate the relief valve, the pressure in the central chamber should be atmospheric. If the inlet pressure should become less than atmospheric pressure, relief valve 3 should remain fully open to the atmosphere to discharge any water which may be caused to backflow as a result of backpressure and leakage of check valve 2.

Malfunctioning of one or both of the check valves or relief valve should always be indicated by a discharge of water from the relief port. Under no circumstances should plugging of the relief port be permitted because the device depends upon an open port for safe operation. The pressure loss through the device may be expected to average between 10 and 20 psi within the normal range of operation, depending upon the size and flow rate of the device.

Reduced pressure principle backflow preventers are commonly installed on high hazard installations such as plating plants, where they would protect against primarily backsiphonage potential, car washes where they would protect against backpressure conditions, and funeral parlors, hospital autopsy rooms, etc. The reduced pressure principle backflow preventer forms the backbone of cross-connection control programs. Since it is utilized to protect against high hazard installations, and since high hazard installations are the first consideration in protecting public health and safety, these devices are installed in large quantities over a broad range of plumbing and water works installations. Figures 31 and 32 show typical installations of these devices on high hazard installations.

FIGURE 30.
Reduced pressure zone backflow preventer — principle of operation.

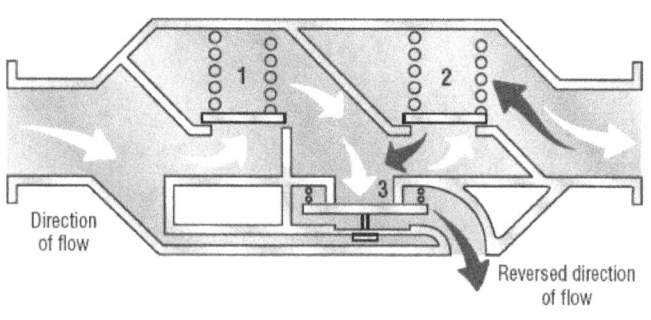

FIGURE 31.
Plating plant installation.

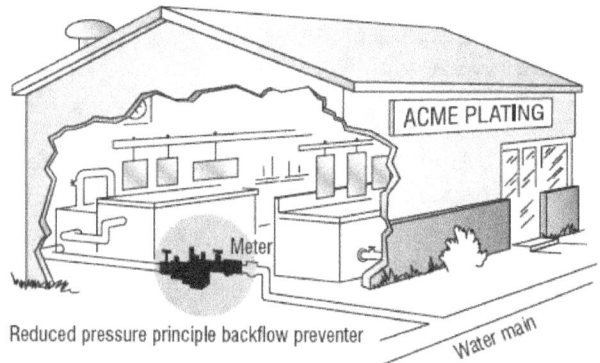

Reduced pressure principle backflow preventer

FIGURE 32.
Car wash installation.

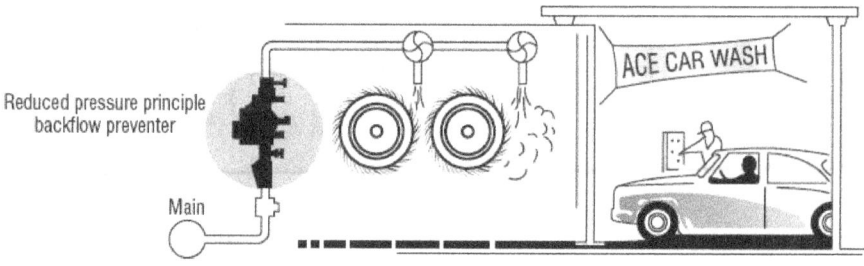

FIGURE 33.
Typical bypass configuration reduced pressure principle devices

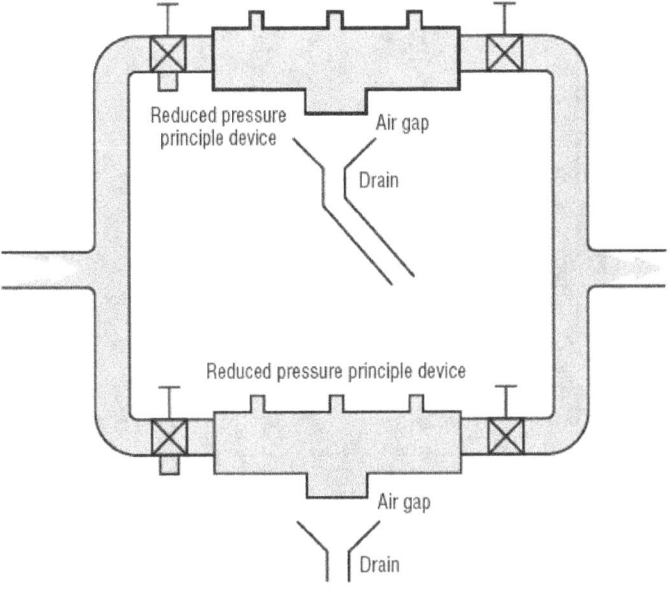

Note: Devices to be set a min. of 12" and a max. of 30' from the floor and 12' from any wall.

Typical fire line installation double check valve vertical installation.

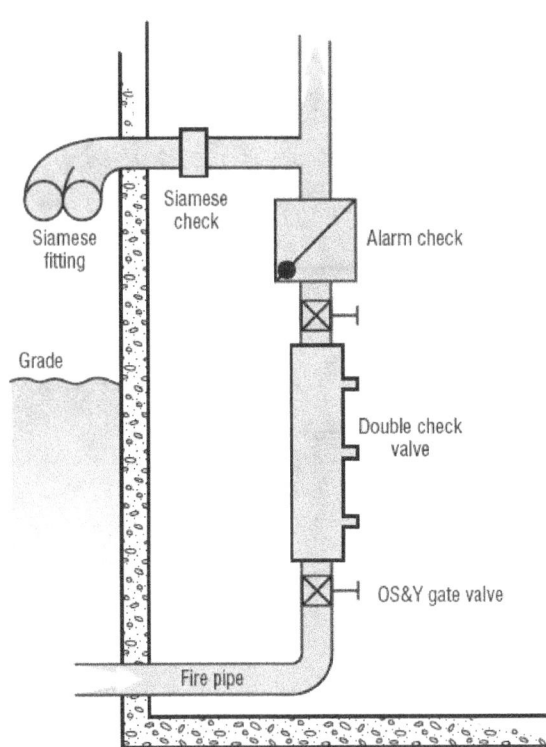

FIGURE 34.
Typical installation reduced pressure principle device horizontal illustration.

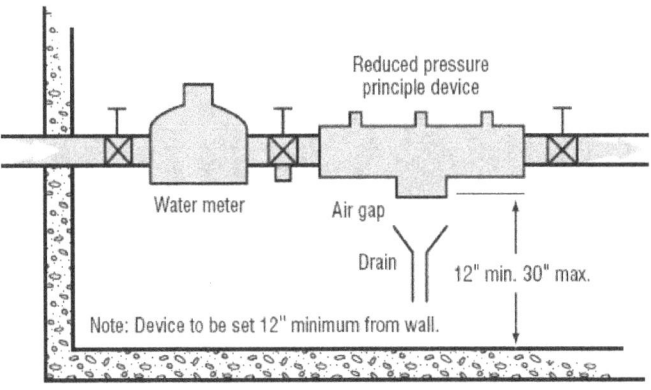

FIGURE 35.
Typical installation reduced pressure principle device vertical illustration.

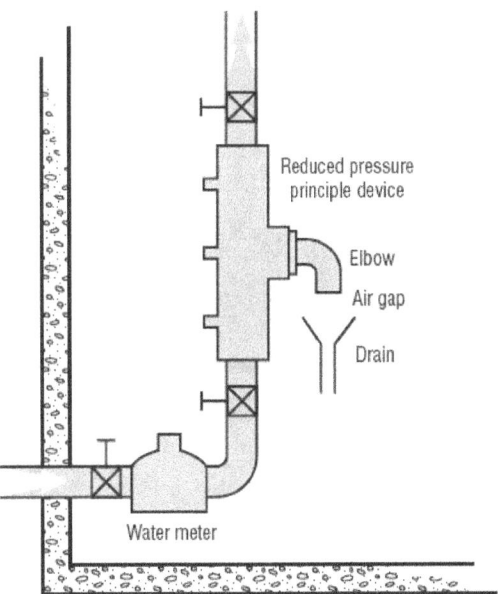

Note: (1) Refer to manufacturers installation data for vertical mount.
(2) Unit to be set at a height to permit ready access for testing and service.
(3) Vertical installation only to be used if horizontal installation cannot be achieved.

FIGURE 36.
Typical installation double check
valve horizontal and vertical
installation.

FIGURE 37.
Typical installation residential dual
check with straight set and
copperhorn.

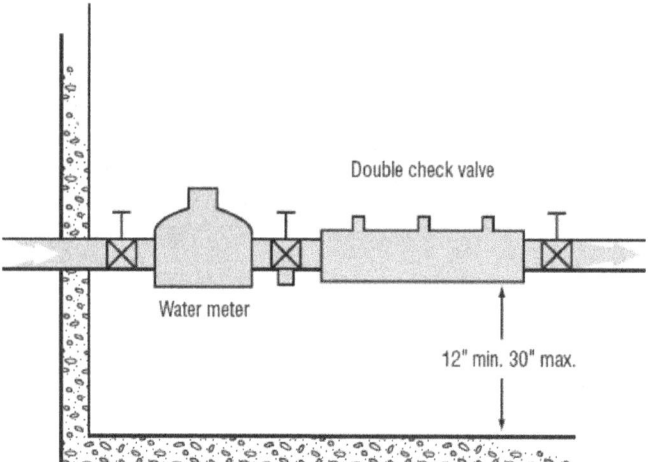

Double check valve

Water meter

12" min. 30" max.

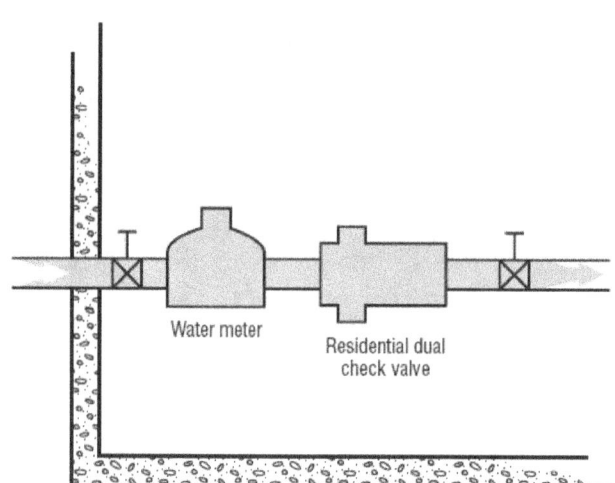

Water meter

Residential dual
check valve

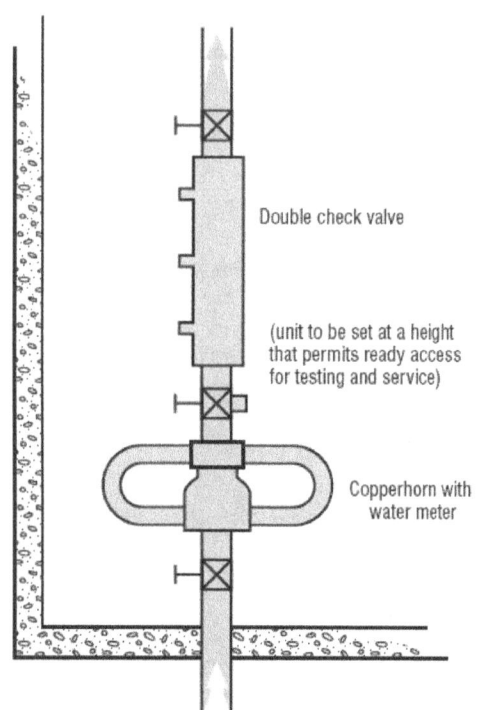

Double check valve

(unit to be set at a height
that permits ready access
for testing and service)

Copperhorn with
water meter

Note: Vertical installation only to be used if horizontal
installation cannot be achieved.

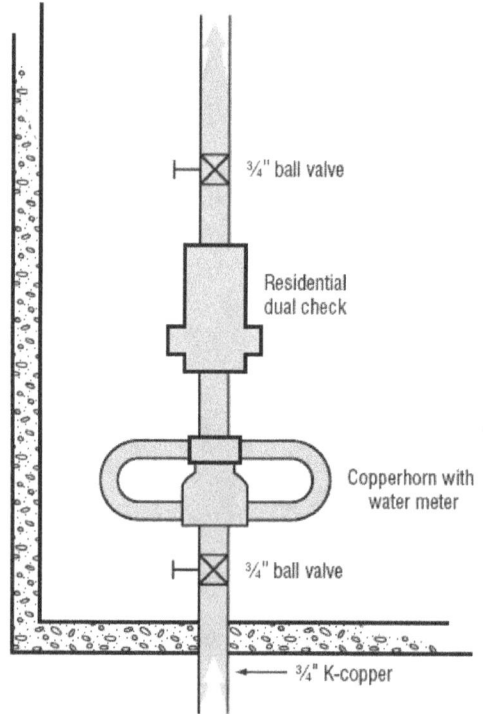

¾" ball valve

Residential
dual check

Copperhorn with
water meter

¾" ball valve

¾" K-copper

Chapter Five

Testing Procedures for Backflow Preventers

Prior to initiating a test of any backflow device, it is recommended that the following procedures be followed:

1. Permission be obtained from the owner, or his representative, to shut down the water supply. This is necessary to insure that since all testing is accomplished under no-flow conditions, the owner is aware that his water supply will be temporarily shut off while the testing is being performed. Some commercial and industrial operations require constant and uninterrupted water supplies for cooling, boiler feed, seal pump water, etc. and water service interruption cannot be tolerated. The water supply to hospitals and continuous process industries cannot be shut off without planned and coordinated shut downs. The request to shut down the water supply is therefore a necessary prerequisite to protect the customer as well as limit the liability of the tester.

Concurrent with the request for permission to shut off the water, it is advisable to point out to the owner, or his representative, that while the water is shut off during the test period, any inadvertent use of water within the building will reduce the water pressure to zero. Backsiphonage could result if unprotected cross-connections existed which would contaminate the building water supply system. In order to address this situation, it is recommended that the owner caution the inhabitants of the building not to use the water until the backflow test is completed and the water pressure restored. Additional options available to the building owner would be the installation of two backflow devices in parallel that would enable a protected bypass flow around the device to be tested. Also, if all water outlets are protected within the building with "fixture outlet protection" backflow devices, cross-connections would not create a problem in the event of potential backsiphonage conditions occurring while devices are tested, or for any other reason.

2. Determine the type of device to be tested i.e., double check valve or reduced pressure principle device.

3. Determine the flow direction. (Reference directional flow arrows or wording provided by the manufacturer on the device.)

4. Number the test cocks, bleed them of potential debris, and assemble appropriate test cock adapters and bushings that may be required.

5. Shut off the downstream (number 2) shut-off valve. (Ref. Item (1) above.)

6. Wait several moments prior to hooking up the test kit hoses when testing a reduced pressure principle device. If water exits the relief valve, in all likelihood, the first check valve is fouled and it is impractical to proceed with the testing until the valve is serviced. This waiting period is not necessary when testing double check valves.

7. Hook up the test kit hoses in the manner appropriate to the device being tested and the specific test being performed.

Test personnel are cautioned to be aware and follow local municipal, county, and state testing requirements and guidelines as may be dictated by local authority. The following test procedures are guidelines for standard, generally acceptable test procedures but may be amended, superceded, or modified by local jurisdiction.

Test Equipment

For field testing of reduced pressure principle backflow preventers and double check valve assemblies, a differential pressure test gauge is utilized having a 0 to 15 psi range and a working pressure of 500 psi. Appropriate length of hoses with necessary fittings accompany the test gauge. Several manufactured test kits are commercially available that incorporate the differential gauge, hoses, and fittings and are packaged for ease of portability and come with protective enclosures or straps for hanging. Calibrated water columns are commercially available that are portable and come with carrying cases.

It is important that all test equipment be periodically checked for calibration.

Pressure Vacuum Breaker

(Figure 38)

Field testing of a pressure vacuum breaker involves testing both the internal spring loaded soft seated check valve as well as testing the spring loaded air inlet valve. The testing must be performed with the device pressurized and the air inlet closed. The number 2 shut-off valve must also be closed and the air inlet valve canopy removed.

Method 1

Using a differential pressure gauge

Test 1 Test the internal check valve for tightness of 1 psid in the direction of flow.

1. With the valve body under pressure, (number 2 shut-off valve closed and

FIGURE 38.

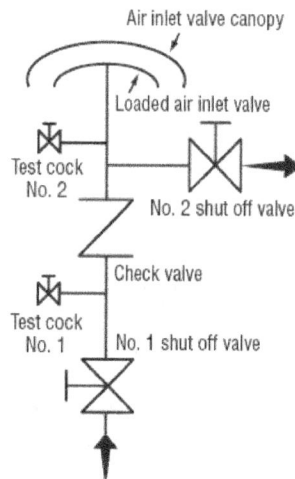

number 1 shut-off valve open) bleed test cocks number 1 and number 2.

2. Hook up the high pressure hose to number 1 test cock and the low pressure hose to number 2 test cock.

3. Bleed the high pressure hose, and low pressure hose, in that order, and close the test kit needle valves slowly.

4. Record the differential pressure on the gauge. A reading of 1 psid is acceptable to insure a tight check valve.

Test 2 Test the air inlet valve for a breakaway of 1 psi.

1. Connect the high pressure hose to test cock number 2, and bleed the high pressure hose.

2. Shut off number 1 shut-off valve.

3. Slowly open the bleed valve of the test kit, and observe and record the psi when the air inlet poppet opens. This should be a minimum of 1 psi. Restore the valve to normal service.

Method 2

Using a water column sight tube and 90 degree elbow fitting with bleed needle

Test 1 Test the internal check valve for tightness of 1 psid in the direction of flow.

1. Assemble sight tube to test cock number 1. Open test cock and fill the tube to a minimum of 36-inches of water height.

2. Close number 1 shut-off valve.

3. Open test cock number 2. The air inlet valve should open and discharge water through number 2 test cock.

4. Open number 1 test cock. The sight tube level of water should drop slowly until it stabilizes. This point should be a minimum of 28-inches of water column which equals 1 psi.

Test 2 Test the air inlet valve for a breakaway of 1 psi.

1. Assemble sight tube to test cock number 2. Open test cock number 2 and fill the tube to a minimum of 36-inches of water height.

2. Close number 1 shut-off valve.

3. Bleed water slowly from the number 2 test cock bleed needle and observe the water column height as it drops.

4. At the point when the air inlet valve pops open, record the height of the water column. This point should be a minimum of 28-inches of water column which equals 1psi.

Restore the valve to normal service.

Reduced Pressure Principle Backflow Preventer

(Figure 39)

Field testing of a reduced pressure principle backflow preventer is accomplished utilizing a differential pressure gauge. The device is tested for three optional characteristics: i.e., (1) the first check valve is tight and maintains a minimum of 5 psi differential pressure, (2) the second check valve is tight against backpressure and (3) the relief valve opens at a minimum of 2 psi below inlet supply pressure. Testing is performed as follows:

Step 1 Test to insure that the first check valve is tight and maintains a minimum pressure of 5 psi differential pressure.

1. Verify that number 1 shut-off valve is open. Close number 2 shut-off valve. If there is no drainage from the relief valve it is assumed that the first check is tight.

2. Close all test kit valves.

3. Connect the high pressure hose to test cock number 2.

4. Connect the low pressure hose to test cock number 3.

5. Open test cocks number 2 and number 3.

6. Open high side bleed needle valve on test kit bleeding the air from the high hose. Close the high side bleed needle valve.

7. Open the low side bleed needle valve on test kit bleeding air from the low hose. Close the low side bleed needle valve. Record the differential gauge pressure. It should be a minimum of 5 psid.

FIGURE 39.

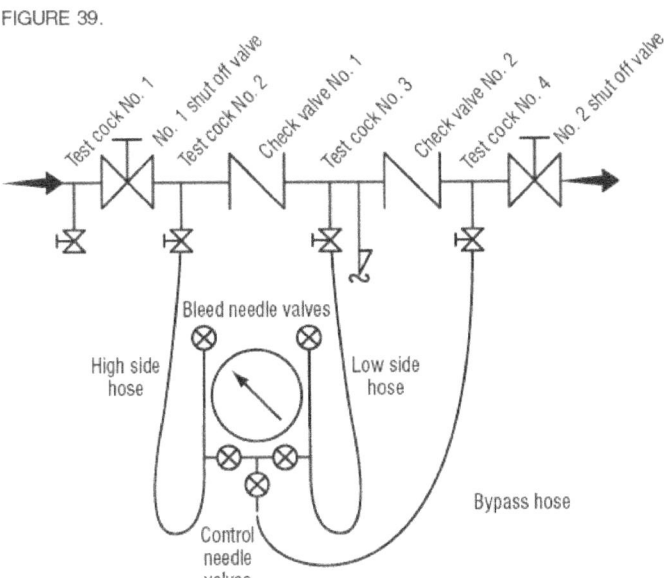

Test cock No. 1
No. 1 shut off valve
Test cock No. 2
Check valve No. 1
Test cock No. 3
Check valve No. 2
Test cock No. 4
No. 2 shut off valve

Bleed needle valves

High side hose

Low side hose

Bypass hose

Control needle valves

Step 2 Test to insure that the second check is tight against backpressure. (Figure 40)

1. Leaving the hoses hooked up as in the conclusion of Step 1 above, connect the bypass hose to test cock number 4.

2. Open test cock number 4, the high control needle valve and the bypass hose control needle valve on the test kit. (This supplies high pressure water downstream of check valve number 2.) If the differential pressure gauge falls off and water comes out of the relief valve, the second check is recorded as leaking. If the differential pressure gauge remains steady, and no water comes out of the relief valve, the second check valve is considered tight

FIGURE 40.

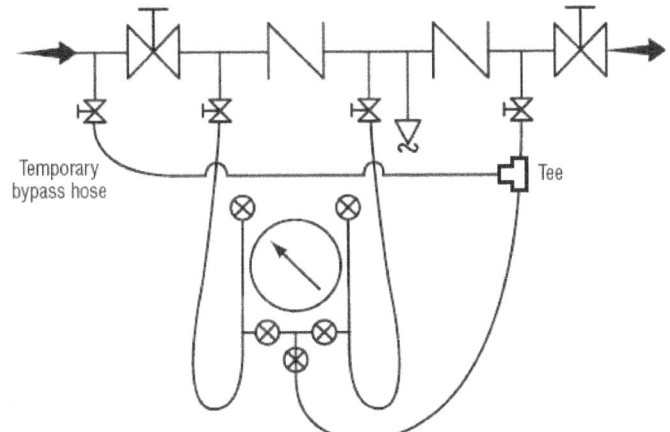

Temporary bypass hose

Tee

3. To check the tightness of number 2 shut-off valve, leave the hoses hooked up the same as at the conclusion of Step 2 above, and then close test cock number 2. This stops the supply of any high pressure water downstream of check valve number 2. If the differential pressure gauge reading holds steady, the number 2 shut-off valve is recorded as being tight. If the differential pressure gauge drops to zero, the number 2 shut-off valve is recorded as leaking.

With a leaking number 2 shut-off valve, the device is, in most cases, in a flow condition and the previous readings taken are invalid. Unless a non-flow condition can be achieved, either through the operation of an additional shut-off downstream, or the use of a temporary compensating bypass hose, accurate test results will not be achieved.

Step 3 To check that the relief valve opens at a minimum pressure of 2 psi below inlet pressure.

1. With the hoses hooked up the same as at the conclusion of Step #2 (3) above, slowly open up the low control needle valve on the test kit and record the differential pressure gauge reading at the point when the water initially starts to drip from the relief valve opening. This pressure reading should not be below 2 psid.

This completes the standard field test for a reduced pressure principle backflow preventer. Before removal of the test equipment, the tester should insure that he opens number 2 shut-off valve thereby reestablishing flow. Also, the test kit should be thoroughly drained of all water to prevent freezing by opening all control needle valves and bleed needle valves.

All test data should be recorded on appropriate forms. (Ref: sample Page 45)

Note: The steps outlined above may vary in sequence depending upon local regulations and/or preferences.

Double Check Valve Assemblies

(Figure 41)
Some field test procedures for testing double check valve assemblies require that the number 1 shut-off valve be closed to accomplish the test. This procedure may introduce debris such as rust and tuberculin into the valve that will impact against check valve number 1 or number 2 and compromise the sealing quality. This potential problem should be considered prior to the selection of the appropriate test method.

Two test methods, one requiring closing of the number 1 shut-off valve, and one without this requirement are presented below:

Method 1

Utilizing the differential pressure gauge and not shutting off number 1 shut-off valve. Figure 41)

Step 1 checking check valve number 1

1. Verify that the number 1 shut-off is open. Shut off number 2 shut-off valve.

2. Connect the high hose to test cock number 2.

3. Connect the low hose to test cock number 3.

4. Open test cocks 2 and 3.

5. Open high side bleed needle valve on test kit bleeding the air from the high hose. Close the high side bleed needle valve.

6. Open low side bleed needle valve on test kit bleeding the air from the low hose. Close the low side bleed needle valve.

FIGURE 41.

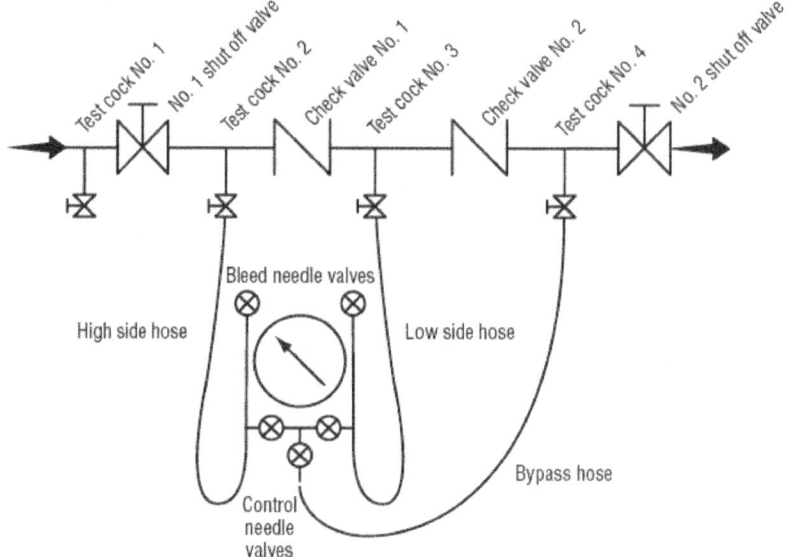

7. Record the differential gauge pressure reading. It should be a minimum of 1 psid.

8. Disconnect the hoses.

Step 2 Checking check valve number 2.

1. Connect the high hose to test cock number 3.

2. Connect the low hose to test cock number 4.

3. Open test cocks number 3 and 4.

4. Open high side bleed needle valve on test kit bleeding the air from the high hose. Close the high side bleed needle valve.

5. Open low side bleed needle valve on test kit bleeding the air from the low hose. Close the low side bleed needle valve.

6. Record the differential gauge pressure reading. It should be a minimum of 1 psid.

7. Disconnect the hoses.

To check tightness of number 2 shut-off valve, both the check valves must be tight and holding a minimum of 1 psid. Also, little or no fluctuation of inlet supply pressure can be tolerated.

The testing is performed as follows:

1. Connect the high hose to number 2 test cock.

2. Connect the low hose to number 3 test cock.

3. Connect the bypass hose to number 4 test cock.

4. Open test cocks numbers 2, 3, and 4.

5. Open high side bleed needle valve on test kit bleeding the air from the high hose. Close the high side bleed needle valve.

6. Open low side bleed needle valve on test kit bleeding the air from the low hose. Close the low side bleed needle valve.

7. The differential gauge pressure should read a minimum of 1 psid.

8. Open the high side control needle valve and the bypass hose control needle valve on the test kit. (This supplies high pressure water downstream of check valve number 2).

9. Close test cock number 2. (This stops the supply of any high pressure water downstream of number 2 check valve), If the differential pressure gauge holds steady, the number 2 shut-off valve is recorded as being tight. If the differential pressure gauge drops to zero, the number 2 shut-off valve is recorded as leaking.

FIGURE 42.

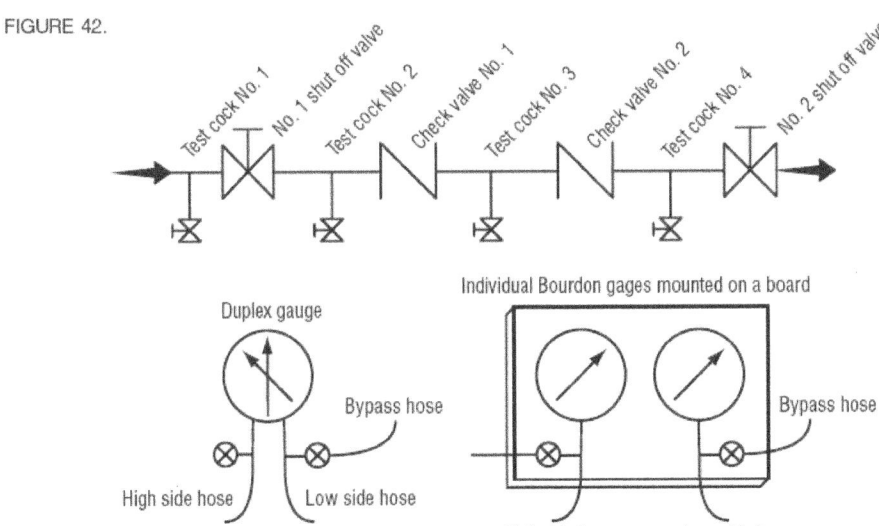

With a leaking number 2 shut-off valve, the device is, in most cases, in a flow condition, and the previous test readings taken are invalid. Unless a non-flow condition can be achieved, either through the operation of an additional shut-off down-stream, or the use of a temporary compensating bypass hose, accurate test results will not be achieved.

This completes the standard field test for a double check valve assembly. Prior to removal of the test equipment, the tester should insure that he opens number 2 shut-off valve thereby reestablishing flow. All test data should be recorded on appropriate forms and the test kit drained of water.

Method 2

Utilizing "Duplex Gauge" or individual bourdon gauges, requires closing number 1 shut-off. (Figure 42)

Step 1 checking check valve number 1

1. Connect the high hose to test cock number 2.

2. Connect the low hose to test cock number 3.

3. Open test cocks number 2 and number 3.

4. Close number 2 shut-off valve; then close number 1 shut-off valve.

5. By means of the high side needle valve, lower the pressure at test cock number 2 about 2 psi below the pressure at test cock number 3. If this small difference can be maintained, then check valve number 1 is reported as "tight". Proceed to Step number 2. If the small difference cannot be maintained, proceed to Step number 3.

Step 2 checking check valve number 2.

Proceed exactly the same test procedure as in Step number 1, except that the high hose is connected to test cock number 3 and the low hose connected to test cock number 4.

Step 3

1. Open shut-off valve number 1 to repressurize the assembly.

2. Loosely attach the bypass hose to test cock number 1, and bleed from the gauge through the bypass hose by opening the low side needle valve to eliminate trapped air. Close low side needle valve. Tighten bypass hose. Open test cock number 1.

3. Close number 1 shut-off valve.

4. By loosening the low side hose at test cock number 3, lower the pressure in the assembly about 10 psi below normal line conditions.

5. Simultaneously open both needle valves. If the check valve is holding tight the high pressure gauge will begin to drop while the low pressure gauge will increase. Close needle valves. If the gauge shows that a small (no more than 5 psi) backpressure is created and held, then the check valve is reported as tight. If the check valve leaks, a pressure differential is not maintained as both gauges tend to equalize or move back towards each other, then the check valve is reported as leaking. With both needle valves open enough to keep the needles on the gauge stationary, the amount of leakage is visible as the discharge from the upstream needle valve.

Chapter Six

Responsibility

Administration of a Cross-Connection Control Program

Under the provisions of the Safe Drinking Water Act of 1974, the Federal Government has established, through the EPA (Environmental Protection Agency), national standards of safe drinking water. The states are responsible for the enforcement of these standards as well as the supervision of public water supply systems and the sources of drinking water. The water purveyor (supplier) is held responsible for compliance to the provisions of the Safe Drinking Water Act, to include a warranty that water quality provided by his operation is in conformance with the EPA standards at the source, and is delivered to the customer without the quality being compromised as a result of its delivery through the distribution system. As specified in the Code of Federal Regulations (Volume 40, Paragraph 141.2, Section (c)) "Maximum contaminant level, means the maximum permissible level of a contaminant in water which is delivered to the free flowing outlet of the ultimate user of a public water system, except in the case of turbidity where the maximum permissible level is measured at the point of entry to the distribution system. Contaminants added to the water under circumstances controlled by the user, except those resulting from corrosion of piping and plumbing caused by water quality, are excluded from this definition."

Figure 43 depicts several options that are open to a water purveyor when considering cross-connection protection to commercial, industrial, and residential customers. He may elect to work initially on the

"containment" theory. This approach utilizes a minimum of backflow devices and isolates the customer from the water main. It virtually insulates the customer from potentially contaminating or polluting the public water supply system. While it is recognized that "containment" does not protect the customer within his building, it does effectively remove him from possible contamination to the public water supply system. If the water purveyor elects to protect his customers on a domestic internal protective basis and/or "fixture outlet protective basis," then cross-connection control protective devices are placed at internal high hazard locations as well as at all locations where cross-connections exist at the "last free-flowing outlet." This approach entails extensive cross-connective survey work on behalf of the water superintendent as well as constant policing of the plumbing within each commercial, industrial and residential account. In large water supply systems, fixture outlet protection cross-connection control philosophy, in itself, is a virtual impossibility to achieve and police due to the quantity of systems involved, the complexity of the plumbing systems inherent in many industrial sites, and the fact that many plumbing changes are made within industrial and commercial establishments that do not require the water department to license or otherwise endorse or ratify when contemplated or completed.

In addition, internal plumbing cross-connection control survey work is generally foreign to the average water

FIGURE 43.

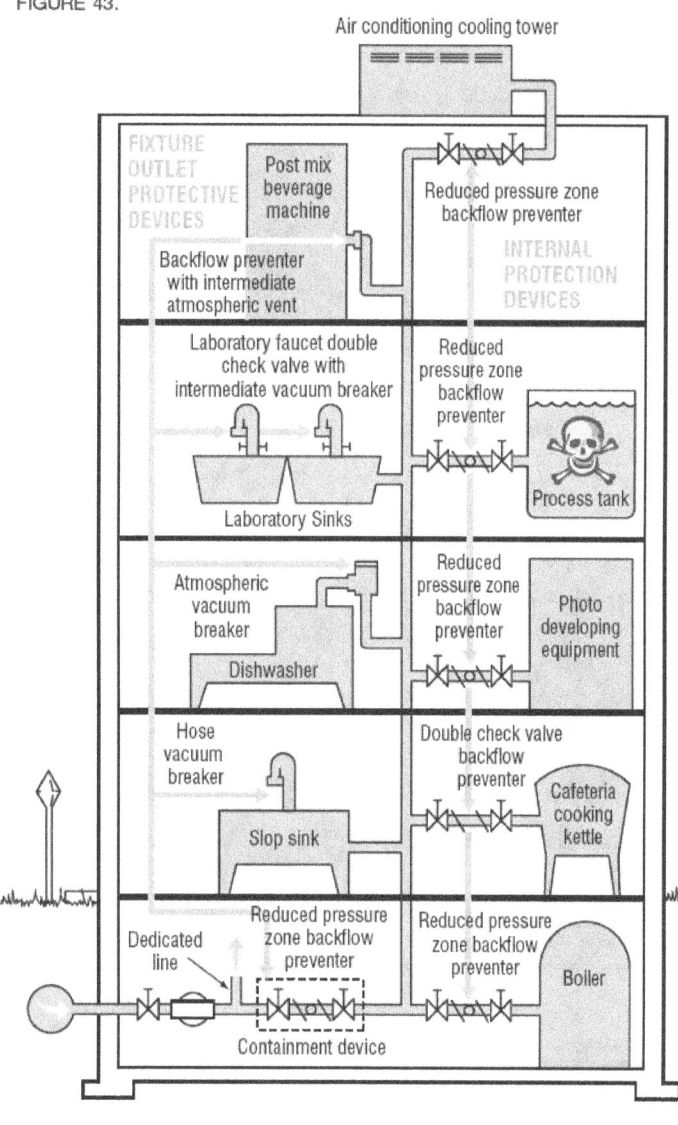

purveyor and is not normally a portion of his job description or duties. While it is admirable for the water purveyor to accept and perform survey work, he should be aware that he runs the risk of additional liability in an area that may be in conflict with plumbing inspectors, maintenance personnel and other public health officials.

Even where extensive "fixture outlet protection," cross-connection control programs are in effect through the efforts of an aggressive and thorough water supply cross-connection control program, the water authorities should also have an active "containment" program in order to address the many plumbing changes that are made and that are inherent within commercial and industrial establishments. In essence, fixture outlet protection becomes an extension beyond the "containment" program.

Also, in order for the supplier of water to provide maximum protection of the water distribution system, consideration should be given to requiring the owner of a premise (commercial, industrial, or residential) to provide at his own expense, adequate proof that his internal water system complies with the local or state plumbing code(s). In addition, he may be required to install, have tested, and maintain, all backflow protection devices that would be required—at his own expense!

The supplier of water should have the right of entry to determine degree of hazard and the existence of cross-connections in order to protect the potable water system. By so doing he can assess the overall

nature of the facility and its potential impact on the water system (determine degree of hazard), personally see actual cross-connections that could contaminate the water system, and take appropriate action to insure the elimination of the cross-connection or the installation of required backflow devices.

To assist the water purveyor in the total administration of a cross-connection control program requires that all public health officials, plumbing inspectors, building managers, plumbing installers, and maintenance men participate and share in the responsibility to protect the public health and safety of individuals from cross-connections and contamination or pollution of the public water supply system.

Dedicated Line

Figure 43 also depicts the use of a "dedicated" potable water line. This line initiates immediately downstream of the water meter and is "dedicated" solely for human consumption i.e., drinking fountains, safety showers, eye wash stations, etc. It is very important that this piping be color coded throughout in accordance with local plumbing regulations, flow direction arrows added, and the piping religiously policed to insure that no cross-connections to other equipment or piping are made that could compromise water quality. In the event that it is felt that policing of this line cannot be reliably maintained or enforced, the installation of a containment device on this line should be a consideration.

A complete cross-connection control program requires a carefully planned and executed initial action plan followed by aggressive implementation and constant follow-up. Proper staffing and education of personnel is a requirement to insure that an effective program is achieved. A recommended plan of action for a cross-connection control program should include the following characteristics:

(1) Establish a cross-connection control ordinance at the local level and have it approved by the water commissioners, town manager, etc., and insure that it is adopted by the town or private water authority as a legally enforceable document.

(2) Conduct public informative meetings that define the proposed cross-connection control program, review the local cross-connection control ordinance, and answer all questions that may arise concerning the reason for the program, why and how the survey will be conducted, and the potential impact upon the industrial, commercial and residential water customers. Have state authorities and the local press and radio attend the meeting.

(3) Place written notices of the pending cross-connection control program in the local newspaper, and have the local radio station make announcements about the program as a public service notice.

(4) Send employees who will administer the program, to a course, or courses, on backflow tester certification, backflow survey courses, backflow device repair courses, etc.

(5) Equip the water authority with backflow device test kits.

(6) Conduct meeting(s) with the local plumbing inspection people, building inspectors, and licensed plumbers in the area who will be active in the inspection, installations and repair of backflow devices. Inform them of the intent of the program and the part that they can play in the successful implementation of the program.

(7) Prior to initiating a survey of the established commercial and industrial installations, prepare a list of these establishments from existing records, then prioritize the degree of hazard that they present to the water system, i.e., plating plants, hospitals, car wash facilities, industrial metal finishing and fabrication, mortuaries, etc. These will be the initial facilities inspected for cross-connections and will be followed by less hazardous installations.

(8) Insure that any new construction plans are reviewed by the water authority to assess the degree of hazard and insure that the proper backflow preventer is installed concurrent with the potential degree of hazard that the facility presents.

(9) Establish a residential backflow protection program that will automatically insure that a residential dual check backflow device is installed automatically at every new residence.

(10) As water meters are repaired or replaced at residences, insure that a residential dual check backflow preventer is set with the new or reworked water meter. Be sure to have the owner address thermal expansion provisions.

Cross-Connection Control Survey Work

(11) Prepare a listing of all testable backflow devices in the community and insure that they are tested by certified test personnel at the time intervals consistent with the local cross-connection control ordinance.

(12) Prepare and submit testing documentation of backflow devices to the State authority responsible for monitoring this data.

(13) Survey all commercial and industrial facilities and require appropriate backflow protection based upon the containment philosophy and/or internal protection and fixture outlet protection. Follow up to insure that the recommended devices are installed and tested on both an initial basis and a periodic basis consistent with the cross-connection control ordinance.

The surveys should be conducted by personnel experienced in commercial and industrial processes. The owners or owners representatives, should be questioned as to what the water is being used for in the facility and what hazards the operations may present to the water system (both within the facility and to the water distribution system) in the event that a backsiphonage or backpressure condition were to exist concurrent with a non-protected cross-connection. In the event that experienced survey personnel are not available within the water authority to conduct the survey, consideration should be given to having a consulting firm perform the survey on behalf of the water department.

Cross-connection control survey work should only be performed by personnel knowledgeable about commercial and industrial potential cross-connections as well as general industrial uses for both potable and process water. If "containment" is the prime objective of the survey, then only sufficient time need be spent in the facility to determine the degree of hazard inherent within the facility or operation. Once this is determined, a judgment can be made by the cross-connection control inspector as to what type of backflow protective device will be needed at the potable supply entrance, or immediately downstream of the water meter. In the event that the cross-connection control program requires "total" protection to the last free flowing outlet, then the survey must be conducted in depth to visually inspect for all cross-connections within the facility and make recommendations and requirements for fixture outlet protective devices, internal protective devices, and containment devices.

It is recommended that consideration be given to the following objectives when performing a cross-connection control survey:

(1) Determine if the survey will be conducted with a pre-arranged appointment or unannounced.

(2) Upon entry, identify yourself and the purpose of the visitation and request to see the plant manager, owner, or maintenance supervisor in order to explain the purpose of the visit and why the cross-connection survey will be of benefit to him.

(3) Ask what processes are involved within the facility and for what purpose potable water is used, i.e., do the boilers have chemical additives? Are air conditioning cooling towers in use with chemical additives? Do they use water savers with chemical additives? Do they have a second source of water (raw water from wells, etc.) in addition to the potable water supply? Does the process water cross-connect with potentially hazardous chemical etching tanks, etc.?

(4) Request "as-built" engineering drawings of the potable water supply in order to trace out internal potable lines and potential areas of cross-connections.

(5) Initiate the survey by starting at the potable entrance supply (the water meter in most cases) and then proceed with the internal survey in the event that total internal protective devices and fixture outlet protective devices are desired.

(6) Survey the plant facilities with the objective of looking for cross-connections at all potable water outlets such as:

> Hose bibbs
> Slop sinks
> Wash room facilities
> Cafeteria and kitchens
> Fire protection and
>   Siamese outlets
> Irrigation outlets
> Boiler rooms
> Mechanical room
> Laundry facilities
>   (hospitals)
> Production floor

(7) Make a sketch of all areas requiring backflow protection devices.

(8) Review with the host what you have found and explain the findings to him. Inform him that he will receive a written report documenting the findings together with a written recommendation for corrective action. Attempt to answer all questions at this time. Review the findings with the owner or manager if time and circumstances permit.

(9) Document all findings and recommendations prior to preparing the written report. Include as many sketches or photos with the final report as possible. If the located cross connection(s) cannot be eliminated, state the generic type of backflow preventer required at each cross connection found.

(10) Consider requiring or recommending compliance of the survey findings within a definitive time frame. (if appropriate authority is in effect).

Chapter Seven

Cross-Connection Control and Backflow Prevention Program

The successful promotion of a cross-connection control and backflow prevention program in a municipality will be dependent upon legal authority to conduct such a program. Where a community has adopted a modern plumbing code, such as the National Plumbing Code, ASA A40.8-1955, or subsequent revisions thereof, provisions of the code will govern backflow and cross-connections. It then remains to provide an ordinance that will establish a program of inspection for an elimination of cross- and backflow connections within the community. Frequently authority for such a program may already be possessed by the water department or water authority. In such cases no further document may be needed. A cross-connection control ordinance should have at least three basic parts.

1. Authority for establishment of a program.
2. Technical provisions relating to eliminating backflow and cross-connections.
3. Penalty provisions for violations.

The following model program is suggested for municipalities who desire to adopt a cross-connection control ordinance. Communities adopting ordinances should check with State health officials to assure conformance with State codes. The form of the ordinance should comply with local legal requirements and receive legal adoption from the community.

CROSS CONNECTION CONTROL MODEL PROGRAM

WATER DEPARTMENT NAME
ADDRESS

DATE

Approved _____

Date _____

Water Department Name
Cross-Connection Control Program

I. **Purpose**

A. To protect the public potable water supply served by the ( ) Water Department from the possibility of contamination or pollution by isolating, within its customers internal distribution system, such contaminants or pollutants which could backflow or back-siphon into the public water system.

B. To promote the elimination or control of existing cross-connections, actual or potential, between its customers in-plant potable water system, and non-potable systems.

C. To provide for the maintenance of a continuing program of cross-connection control which will effectively prevent the contamination or pollution of all potable water systems by cross-connection.

II. **Authority**

A. The Federal Safe Drinking Water Act of 1974, and the statutes of the State of ( ) Chapters ( ) the water purveyor has the primary responsibility for preventing water from unapproved sources, or any other substances, from entering the public potable water system.

B. ( ) Water Department, Rules and Regulations, adopted.

III. Responsibility

The Director of Municipal Services shall be responsible for the protection of the public potable water distribution system from contamination or pollution due to the backflow or backsiphonage of contaminants or pollutants through the water service connection. If, in the judgment of the Director of Municipal Services, an approved backflow device is required at the city's water service connection to any customer's promises, the Director, or his delegated agent, shall give notice in writing to said customer to install an approved backflow prevention device at each service connection to his premises. The customer shall, within 90 days install such approved device, or devices, at his own expense, and failure or refusal, or inability on the part of the customer to install said device or devices within ninety (90) days, shall constitute a ground for discontinuing water service to the premises until such device or devices have been properly installed.

IV. Definitions

A. Approved

Accepted by the Director of Municipal Services as meeting an applicable specification stated or cited in this regulation, or as suitable for the proposed use.

B. Auxiliary Water Supply

Any water supply, on or available, to the premises other than the purveyor's approved public potable water supply.

C. Backflow

The flow of water or other liquids, mixtures or substances, under positive or reduced pressure in the distribution pipes of a potable water supply from any source other than its intended source.

D. Backflow Preventer

A device or means designed to prevent backflow or backsiphonage. Most commonly categorized as air gap, reduced pressure principle device, double check valve assembly, pressure vacuum breaker, atmospheric vacuum breaker, hose bibb vacuum breaker, residential dual check, double check with intermediate atmospheric vent, and barometric loop.

D.1 Air Gap

A physical separation sufficient to prevent backflow between the free-flowing discharge end of the potable water system and any other system. Physically defined as a distance equal to twice the diameter of the supply side pipe diameter but never less than one (1) inch.

D.2 Atmospheric Vacuum Breaker

A device which prevents backsiphonage by creating an atmospheric vent when there is either a negative pressure or subatmospheric pressure in a water system.

D.3 Barometric Loop

A fabricated piping arrangement rising at least thirty five (35) feet at its topmost point above the highest fixture it supplies. It is utilized in water supply systems to protect against backsiphonage.

D.4 Double Check Valve Assembly

An assembly of two (2) independently operating spring loaded check valves with tightly closing shut off valves on each side of the check valves, plus properly located test cocks for the testing of each check valve.

D.5 Double Check Valve with Intermediate Atmospheric Vent

A device having two (2) spring loaded check valves separated by an atmospheric vent chamber.

D.6 Hose Bibb Vacuum Breaker

A device which is permanently attached to a hose bibb and which acts as an atmospheric vacuum breaker.

D.7 Pressure Vacuum Breaker

A device containing one or two independently operated spring loaded check valves and an independently operated spring loaded air inlet valve located on the discharge side of the check or checks. Device includes tightly closing shut-off valves on each side of the check valves and properly located test cocks for the testing of the check valve(s).

D.8 Reduced Pressure Principle Backflow Preventer

An assembly consisting of two (2) independently operating approved check valves with an automatically operating differential relief valve located between the two (2) check valves, tightly closing shut-off valves on each side of the check valves plus properly located test cocks for the testing of the check valves and the relief valve.

D.9 Residential Dual Check

An assembly of two (2) spring loaded, independently operating check valves without tightly closing shut-off valves and test cocks. Generally employed immediately downstream of the water meter to act as a containment device.

E. Backpressure

A condition in which the owners system pressure is greater than the suppliers system pressure.

F. Backsiphonage

The flow of water or other liquids, mixtures or substances into the distribution pipes of a potable water supply system from any source other than its intended source caused by the sudden reduction of pressure in the potable water supply system.

G. Commission

The State of (   ) Control Commission.

H. Containment

A method of backflow prevention which requires a backflow prevention preventer at the water service entrance.

I. Contaminant

A substance that will impair the quality of the water to a degree that it creates a serious health hazard to the public leading to poisoning or the spread of disease.

J. Cross-Connection

Any actual or potential connection between the public water supply and a source of contamination or pollution.

K. Department

City of (   ) Water Department.

L. Fixture Isolation

A method of backflow prevention in which a backflow preventer is located to correct a cross connection at an in-plant location rather than at a water service entrance.

M. Owner

Any person who has legal title to, or license to operate or habitat in, a property upon which a cross-connection inspection is to be made or upon which a cross-connection is present.

N. Person

Any individual, partnership, company, public or private corporation, political subdivision or agency of the State Department, agency or instrumentality or the United States or any other legal entity.

O. Permit

A document issued by the Department which allows the use of a backflow preventer.

P. Pollutant

A foreign substance, that if permitted to get into the public water system, will degrade its quality so as to constitute a moderate hazard, or impair the usefulness or quality of the water to a degree which does not create an actual hazard to the public health but which does adversely and unreasonably effect such water for domestic use.

Q. Water Service Entrance

That point in the owners water system beyond the sanitary control of the District; generally considered to be the outlet end of the water meter and always before any unprotected branch.

R. Director of Municipal Services

The Director, or his delegated representative in charge of the (   ) Department of Municipal Services, is invested with the authority and responsibility for the implementation of a cross-connection control program and for the enforcement of the provisions of the Ordinance.

V. Administration

A. The Department will operate a cross-connection control program, to include the keeping of necessary records, which fulfills the requirements of the Commission's Cross-Connection Regulations and is approved by the Commission.

B. The Owner shall allow his property to be inspected for possible cross-connections and shall follow the provisions of the Department's program and the Commission's Regulations if a cross-connection is permitted.

C. If the Department requires that the public supply be protected by containment, the Owner shall be responsible for water quality beyond the outlet end of the containment device and should utilize fixture outlet protection for that purpose.

He may utilize public health officials, or personnel from the Department, or their delegated representatives, to assist him in the survey of his facilities and to assist him in the selection of proper fixture outlet devices, and the proper installation of these devices.

VI. Requirements

A. Department

1. On new installations, the Department will provide on-site evaluation and/or inspection of plans in order to determine the type of backflow preventer, if any, that will be required, will issue permit, and perform inspection and testing. In any case, a minimum of a dual check valve will be required in any new construction.

2. For premises existing prior to the start of this program, the Department will perform evaluations and inspections of plans and/or premises and inform the owner by letter of any corrective action deemed necessary, the method of achieving the correction, and the time allowed for the correction to be made. Ordinarily, ninety (90) days will be allowed, however, this time period may be shortened depending upon the degree of hazard involved and the history of the device(s) in question.

3. The Department will not allow any cross-connection to remain unless it is protected by an approved backflow preventer for which a permit has been issued and which will be regularly tested to insure satisfactory operation.

4. The Department shall inform the Owner by letter, of any failure to comply, by the time of the first re-inspection. The Department will allow an additional fifteen (15) days for the correction. In the event the Owner fails to comply with the necessary correction by the time of the second re-inspection, the Department will inform the Owner by letter, that the water service to the Owner's premises will be terminated within a period not to exceed five (5) days. In the event that the Owner informs the Department of extenuating circumstances as to why the correction has not been made, a time extension may be granted by the Department but in no case will exceed an additional thirty (30) days.

5. If the Department determines at any time that a serious threat to the public health exists, the water service will be terminated immediately.

6. The Department shall have on file, a list of Private Contractors who are certified backflow device testers. All charges for these tests will be paid by the Owner of the building or property.

7. The Department will begin initial premise inspections to determine the nature of existing or potential hazards, following the approval of this program by the Commission, during the calendar year (   ). Initial focus will be on high hazard industries and commercial premises.

B. Owner

1. The Owner shall be responsible for the elimination or protection of all cross-connections on his premises.

2. The Owner, after having been informed by a letter from the Department, shall at his expense, install, maintain, and test, or have tested, any and all backflow preventers on his premises.

3. The Owner shall correct any malfunction of the backflow preventer which is revealed by periodic testing.

4. The Owner shall inform the Department of any proposed or modified cross-connections and also any existing cross-connections of which the Owner is aware but has not been found by the Department.

5. The Owner shall not install a bypass around any backflow preventer unless there is a backflow preventer of the same type on the bypass. Owners who cannot shut down operation for testing of the device(s) must supply additional devices necessary to allow testing to take place. (Ref. Fig. 33 page 23.)

6. The Owner shall install backflow preventers in a manner approved by the Department. (Ref. Figures 3 through 37, pages 23 through 24.)

7. The Owner shall install only backflow preventers approved by the Department or the Commission.

8. Any Owner having a private well or other private water source, must have a permit if the well or source is cross-connected to the Department's system. Permission to cross-connect may be denied by the Department. The Owner may be required to install a backflow preventer at the service entrance if a private water source is maintained, even if it is not cross-connected to the Department's system.

9. In the event the Owner installs plumbing to provide potable water for domestic purposes which is on the Department's side of the backflow preventer, such plumbing must have its own backflow preventer installed.

10. The Owner shall be responsible for the payment of all fees for permits, annual or semi-annual device testing, retesting in the case that the device fails to operate correctly, and second re-inspections for non-compliance with Department or Commission requirements.

VII. Degree of Hazard

The Department recognizes the threat to the public water system arising from cross-connections. All threats will be classified by degree of hazard and will require the installation of approved reduced pressure principle backflow prevention devices or double check valves.

VIII. Permits

The Department shall not permit a cross-connection within the public water supply system unless it is considered necessary and that it cannot be eliminated.

A. Cross-connection permits that are required for each backflow prevention device are obtained from the Department. A fee of (   ) dollars will be charged for the initial permit and (   ) dollars for the renewal of each permit.

B. Permits shall be renewed every (   ) years and are non-transferable. Permits are subject to revocation and become immediately revoked if the Owner should so change the type of cross-connection or degree of hazard associated with the service.

C. A permit is not required when fixture isolation is achieved with the utilization of a non-testable backflow preventer.

IX. Existing in-use backflow prevention devices.

Any existing backflow preventer shall be allowed by the Department to continue in service unless the degree of hazard is such as to supercede the effectiveness of the present backflow preventer, or result in an unreasonable risk to the public health. Where the degree of hazard has increased, as in the case of a residential installation converting to a business establishment, any existing backflow preventer must be upgraded to a reduced pressure principle device, or a reduced pressure principle device must be installed in the event that no backflow device was present.

X. Periodic Testing

A. Reduced pressure principle backflow devices shall be tested and inspected at least semi-annually.

B. Periodic testing shall be performed by the Department's certified tester or his delegated representative. This testing will be done at the owner's expense.

C. The testing shall be conducted during the Department's regular business hours. Exceptions to this, when at the request of the owner, may require additional charges to cover the increased costs to the Department.

D. Any backflow preventer which fails during a periodic test will be repaired or replaced. When repairs are necessary, upon completion of the repair the device will be re-tested at owners expense to insure correct operation. High hazard situations will not be allowed to continue unprotected if the backflow preventer fails the test and cannot be repaired immediately. In other situations, a compliance date of not more than thirty (30) days after the test date will be established. The owner is responsible for spare parts, repair tools, or a replacement device. Parallel installation of two (2) devices is an effective means of the owner insuring that uninterrupted water service during testing or repair of devices and is strongly recommended when the owner desires such continuity. (Ref. Fig. 33 page 23.)

E. Backflow prevention devices will be tested more frequently than specified in A. above, in cases where there is a history of test failures and the Department feels that due to the degree of hazard involved, additional testing is warranted. Cost of the additional tests will be born by the owner.

XI. Records and Reports

A. Records

The Department will initiate and maintain the following:

1. Master files on customer cross-connection tests and/or inspections.

2. Master files on cross-connection permits.

3. Copies of permits and permit applications.

4. Copies of lists and summaries supplied to the Commission.

B. Reports

The Department will submit the following to the Commission.

1. Initial listing of low hazard cross-connections to the State.

2. Initial listing of high hazard cross-connections to the State.

3. Annual update lists of items 1 and 2 above.

4. Annual summary of cross-connection inspections to the State.

XII. Fees and Charges

The Department will publish a list of fees or charges for the following services or permits:

1. Testing fees

2. Re-testing fees

3. Fee for re-inspection

4. Charges for after-hours inspections or tests.

Addendum

1. **Residential dual check**

Effective the date of the acceptance of this Cross-Connection Control Program for the Town of (   ) all new residential buildings will be required to install a residential dual check device immediately downstream of the water meter. (Ref. Figure 37 page 24.) Installation of this residential dual check device on a retrofit basis on existing service lines will be instituted at a time and at a potential cost to the homeowner as deemed necessary by the Department.

The owner must be aware that installation of a residential dual check valve results in a potential closed plumbing system within his residence. As such, provisions may have to be made by the owner to provide for thermal expansion within his closed loop system, i.e., the installation of thermal expansion devices and/or pressure relief valves.

2. **Strainers**

The Department strongly recommends that all new retrofit installations of reduced pressure principle devices and double check valve backflow preventers include the installation of strainers located immediately upstream of the backflow device. The installation of strainers will preclude the fouling of backflow devices due to both foreseen and unforeseen circumstances occurring to the water supply system such as water main repairs, water main breaks, fires, periodic cleaning and flushing of mains, etc. These occurrences may "stir up" debris within the water main that will cause fouling of backflow devices installed without the benefit of strainers.

Partial List of Plumbing Hazards

Fixtures with Direct Connections

Description

Air conditioning, air washer
Air conditioning, chilled water
Air conditioning, condenser
    water
Air line
Aspirator, laboratory
Aspirator, medical
Aspirator, weedicide and
    fertilizer sprayer
Autoclave and sterilizer
Auxiliary system, industrial
Auxiliary system, surface water
Auxiliary system, unapproved
    well supply
Boiler system
Chemical feeder, pot-type
Chlorinator
Coffee urn
Cooling system
Dishwasher
Fire standpipe or sprinkler
    system
Fountain, ornamental
Hydraulic equipment
Laboratory equipment
Lubrication, pump bearings
Photostat equipment
Plumber's friend, pneumatic
Pump, pneumatic ejector
Pump, prime line
Pump, water operated ejector

Sewer, sanitary
Sewer, storm
Swimming pool

Fixtures with Submerged Inlets

Description

Baptismal fount
Bathtub
Bedpan washer, flushing rim
Bidet
Brine tank
Cooling tower
Cuspidor
Drinking fountain
Floor drain, flushing rim
Garbage can washer
Ice maker
Laboratory sink, serrated nozzle
Laundry machine
Lavatory
Lawn sprinkler system
Photo laboratory sink
Sewer flushing manhole
Slop sink, flushing rim
Slop sink, threaded supply
Steam table
Urinal, siphon jet blowout
Vegetable peeler
Water closet, flush tank,
    ball cock
Water closet, flush valve,
    siphon jet

Illustrations of Backsiphonage

The following illustrates typical plumbing installations where backsiphonage is possible.

Backsiphonage

Case I (Fig. 44)

A. Contact Point: A rubber hose is submerged in a bedpan wash sink.

B. Causes of Reversed Flow: (1) A sterilizer connected to the water supply is allowed to cool without opening the air vent. As it cools, the pressure within the sealed sterilizer drops below atmospheric producing a vacuum which draws the polluted water into the sterilizer contaminating its contents. (2) The flushing of several flush valve toilets on a lower floor which are connected to an undersized water service line reduces the pressure at the water closets to atmospheric producing a reversal of the flow. C. Suggested Correction: The water connection at the bedpan wash sink and the sterilizer should be provided with properly installed backflow preventers.

Backsiphonage

Case 2 (Fig. 45)

A. Contact Point: A rubber hose is submerged in a laboratory sink.

B. Cause of Reversed Flow: Two opposite multi-story buildings are connected to the same water main, which often lacks adequate pressure. The building on the right has installed a booster pump.

FIGURE 44.
Backsiphonage (Case 1).

FIGURE 45.
Backsiphonage (Case 2).

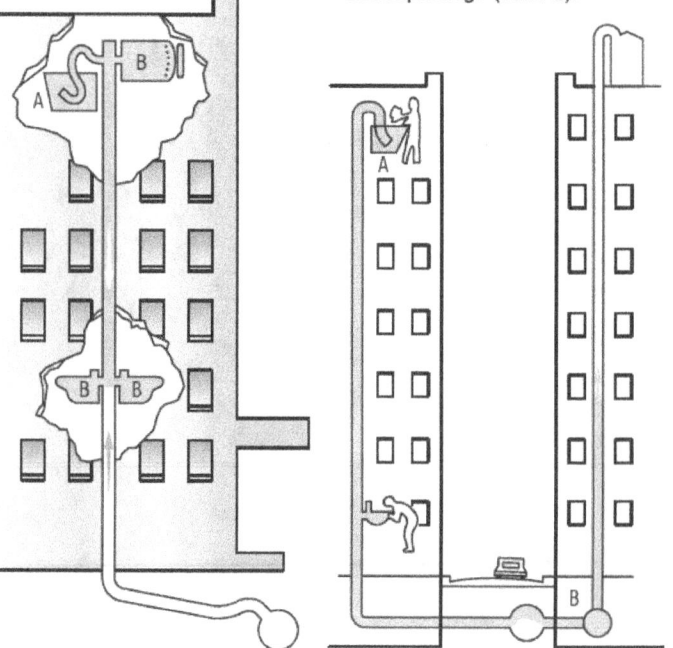

When the pressure is inadequate in the main, the building booster pump starts pumping, producing a negative pressure in the main and causing a reversal of flow in the opposite building.

C. Suggested Correction: The laboratory sink water outlet should be provided with a vacuum breaker. The water service line to the booster pump should be equipped with a device to cut off the pump when pressure approaches a negative head or vacuum.

Backsiphonage

Case 3 (Fig. 46)

A. Contact Point: A chemical tank has a submerged inlet.

B. Cause of Reversed Flow: The plant fire pump draws suction directly from the city water supply line which is insufficient to serve normal plant requirements and a major fire at the same time. During a fire emergency, reversed flow may occur within the plant.

C. Suggested Correction: The water service to the chemical tank should be provided through an air gap.

FIGURE 46.
Backsiphonage (Case 3).

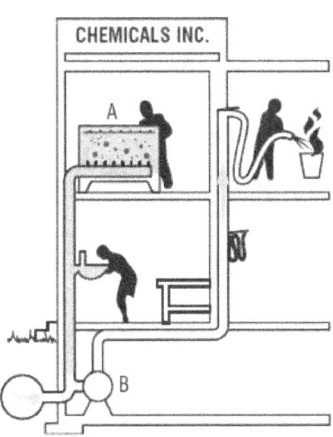

Backsiphonage

Case 4 (Fig. 47)

A. Contact Point: The water supply to the dishwasher is not protected by a vacuum breaker. Also, the dishwasher has a solid waste connection to the sewer.

B. Cause of Reversed Flow: The undersized main serving the building is subject to reduced pressures, and therefore only the first two floors of the building are supplied directly with city pressure. The upper floors are served from a booster pump drawing suction directly from the water service line. During periods of low city pressure, the booster pump suction creates negative pressures in the low system, thereby reversing the flow.

C. Suggested Correction: The dishwasher hot and cold water should be supplied through an air gap and the waste from the dishwasher should discharge through an indirect waste. The booster pump should be equipped with a low-pressure cutoff device.

FIGURE 47.
Backsiphonage (Case 4).

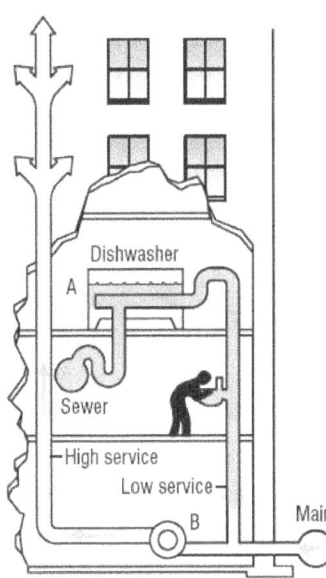

Backsiphonage

Case 5 (Fig. 48)

A. Contact Point: The gasoline storage tank is maintained full and under pressure by means of a direct connection to the city water distribution system.

FIGURE 48.
Backsiphonage (Case 5).

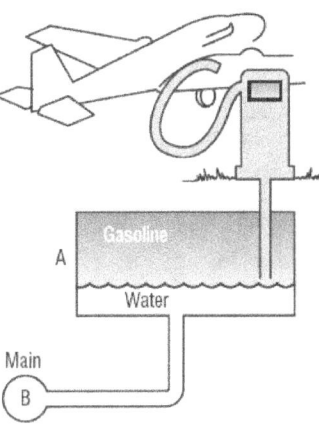

B. Cause of Reversed Flow: Gasoline may enter the distribution system by gravity or by siphonage in the event of a leak or break in the water main.

C. Suggested Correction: A reduced pressure principle backflow preventer should be installed in the line to the gasoline storage tank or a surge tank and pump should be provided in that line.

Backsiphonage

Case 6 (Fig. 49)

A. Contact Point: There is a submerged inlet in the second floor bathtub.

B. Cause of Reversed Flow: An automobile breaks a nearby fire hydrant causing a rush of water and a negative pressure in the service line to the house, sucking dirty water out of the bathtub.

C. Suggested Correction: The hot and cold water inlets to the bathtub should be above the rim of the tub.

FIGURE 49.
Backsiphonage (Case 6).

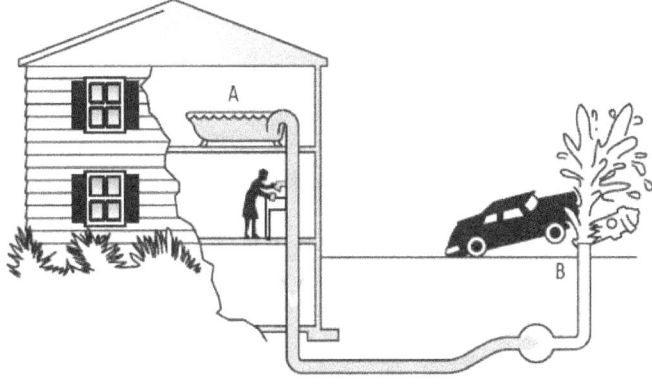

Illustrations of Backpressure

The following presents illustrations of typical plumbing installations where backflow resulting from backpressure is possible.

Backflow

Case I (Fig. 50)

A. Contact Point: A direct connection from the city supply to the boiler exists as a safety measure and for filling the system. The boiler water system is chemically treated for scale prevention and corrosion control.

B. Cause of Reversed Flow: The boiler water recirculation pump discharge pressure or backpressure from the boiler exceeds the city water pressure and the chemically treated water is pumped into the domestic system through an open or leaky valve.

C. Suggested Correction: As minimum protection two check valves in series should be provided in the makeup waterline to the boiler system. An air gap separation or reduced pressure principle backflow preventer is better.

FIGURE 50.
Backflow (Case 1).

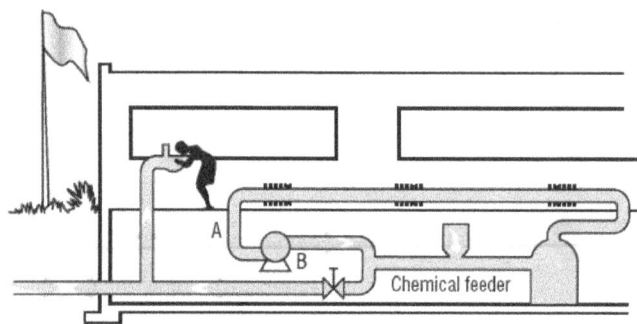

FIGURE 51.
Backflow (Case 2).

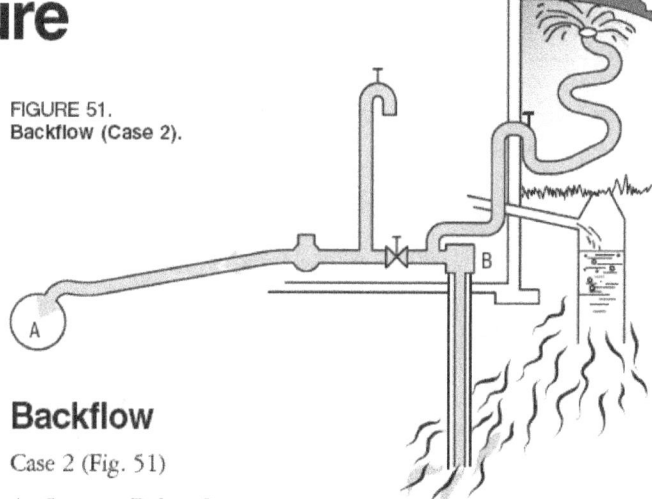

Backflow

Case 2 (Fig. 51)

A. Contact Point: Sewage seeping from a residential cesspool pollutes the private well which is used for lawn sprinkling. The domestic water system, which is served from a city main, is connected to the well supply by means of a valve. The purpose of the connection may be to prime the well supply for emergency domestic use.

B. Cause of Reversed Flow: During periods of low city water pressure, possibly when lawn sprinkling is at its peak, the well pump discharge pressure exceeds that of the city main and well water is pumped into the city supply through an open or leaky valve.

C. Suggested Correction: The connection between the well water and city water should be broken

Backflow

Case 3 (Fig. 52)

A. Contact Point: A valve connection exists between the potable and the non potable systems aboard the ship.

B. Cause of Reversed Flow: While the ship is connected to the city water supply system for the purpose of taking on water for the potable system, the valve between the potable and nonpotable systems is opened, permitting contaminated water to be pumped into the municipal supply.

FIGURE 52.
Backflow (Case 3).

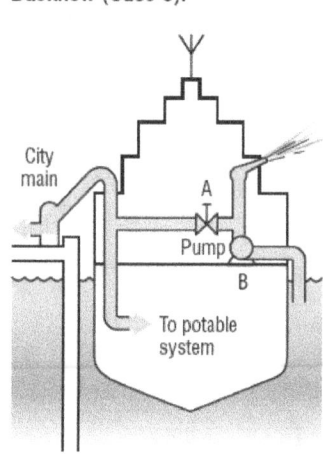

City main

Pump

To potable system

C. Suggested Correction: Each pier water outlet should be protected against backflow. The main water service to the pier should also be protected against backflow by an air gap or reduced pressure principle backflow preventer.

Backflow

Case 4 (Fig. 53)

A. Contact Point: A single-valved connection exists between the public, potable water supply and the fire-sprinkler system of a mill.

B. Cause of Reversed Flow: The sprinkler system is normally supplied from a nearby lake through a high-pressure pump. About the lake are large numbers of overflowing septic tanks. When the valve is left open, contaminated lake water can be pumped to the public supply.

C. Suggested Correction: The potable water supply to the fire system should be through an air gap or a reduced pressure principle backflow preventer should be used.

FIGURE 53.
Backflow (Case 4).

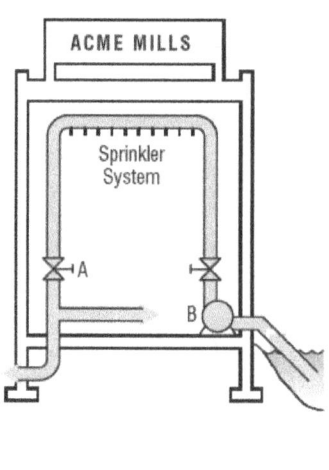

ACME MILLS

Sprinkler System

Illustrations of Air Gaps

The following illustrations describe methods of providing an air gap discharge to a waste line which may be occasionally or continuously subject to backpressure.

FIGURE 54.
Air gap to sewer subject to backpressure—force main.

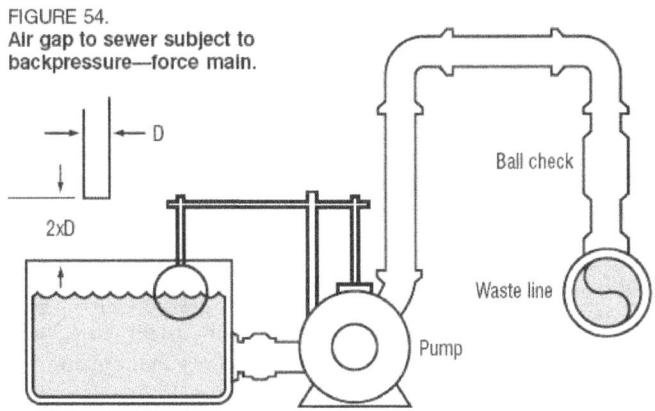

FIGURE 55.
Air gap to sewer subject to backpressure—gravity drain.

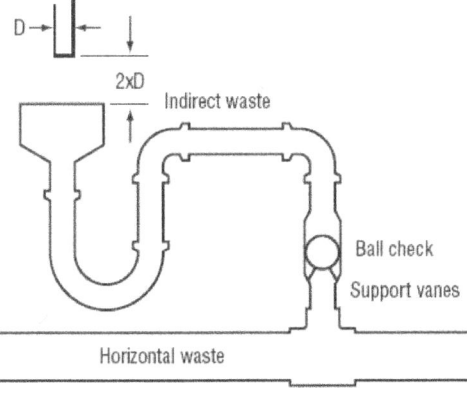

FIGURE 56.
Fire system makeup tank for a dual water system.

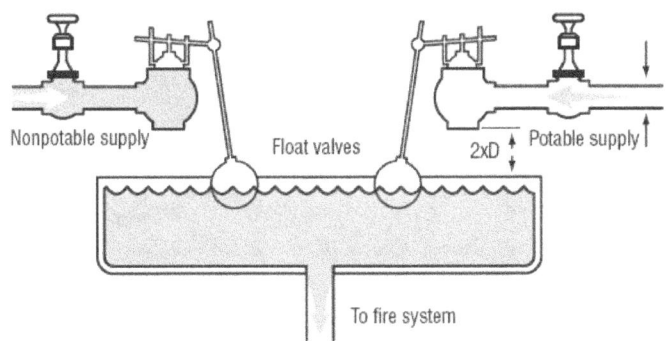

Illustrations of Vacuum Breakers

FIGURE 57.
Vacuum breakers.

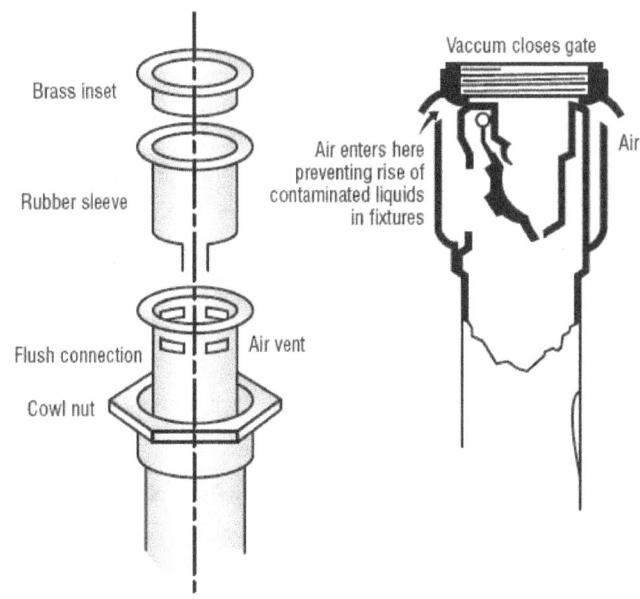

FIGURE 58.
Vacuum breaker arrangement for an outside hose hydrant.

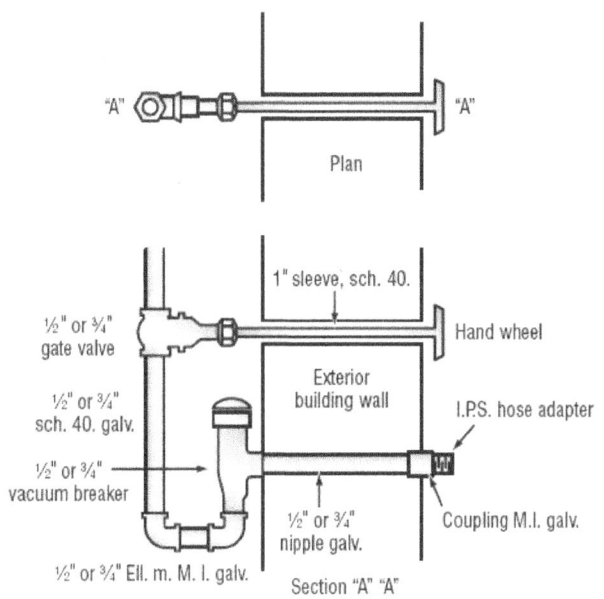

(By permission of Mr. Gustave J. Angele Sr., P.E. formerly Plant Sanitary Engineer, Union Carbide Nuclear Division, Oak Ridge, Tenn.)

Glossary

Air gap The unobstructed vertical distance through the free atmosphere between the lowest opening from any pipe or faucet supplying water to a tank, plumbing fixture, or other device and the flood-level rim of the receptacle.

Backflow The flow of water or other liquids, mixtures, or substances into the distributing pipes of a potable supply of water from any source or sources other than its intended source. Backsiphonage is one type of backflow.

Backflow Connection Any arrangement whereby backflow can occur.

Backflow Preventer A device or means to prevent backflow. Backflow Preventer, Reduced Pressure Principle Type An assembly of differential valves and check valves including an automatically opened spillage port to the atmosphere.

Backsiphonage Backflow resulting from negative pressures in the distributing pipes of a potable water supply.

Cross-Connection Any actual or potential connection between the public water supply and a source of contamination or pollution.

Effective Opening The minimum cross-sectional area at the point of water supply discharge, measured or expressed in terms of (1) diameter of a circle, or (2) if the opening is not circular, the diameter of a circle or equivalent cross-sectional area.

Flood-Level Rim The edge of the receptacle from which water overflows.

Flushometer Valve A device which discharges a predetermined quantity of water to fixtures for flushing purposes and is actuated by direct water pressure.

Free Water Surface A water surface that is at atmospheric pressure.

Frostproof Closet A hopper with no water in the bowl and with the trap and water supply control valve located below frost line.

Indirect Waste Pipe A drain pipe used to convey liquid wastes that does not connect directly with the drainage system, but which discharges into the drainage system through an air break into a vented trap or a properly vented and trapped fixture, receptacle, or interceptor.

Plumbing The practice, materials, and fixtures used in the installation, maintenance, extension, and alteration of all piping, fixtures, appliances and appurtenances in connection with any of the following: sanitary drainage or storm drainage facilities, the venting system and the public or private water-supply systems, within or adjacent to any building, structure, or conveyance; also the practice and materials used in the installation, maintenance, extension, or alteration of storm water, liquid waste, or sewerage, and water-supply systems of any premises to their connection with any point of public disposal or other acceptable terminal.

Potable Water Water free from impurities present in amounts sufficient to cause disease or harmful physiological effects. Its bacteriological and chemical quality shall conform to the requirements of the USEPA National Primary Drinking Water Regulations and the regulations of the public health authority having jurisdiction.

Vacuum Any absolute pressure less than that exerted by the atmosphere.

Vacuum Breaker A device that permits air into a water supply distribution line to prevent backsiphonage.

Water Outlet A discharge opening through which water is supplied to a fixture, into the atmosphere (except into an open tank which is part of the water supply system), to a boiler or heating system, to any devices or equipment requiring water to operate but which are not part of the plumbing system.

Water Supply System The water service pipe, the water-distributing pipes, and the necessary connecting pipes, fittings, control valves, and all appurtenances in or adjacent to the building or premises. The water supply system is part of the plumbing system.

Appendix G

Bibliography

Accepted Procedure and Practice in Cross-Connection Control Manual, American Water Works Association, Pacific Northwest Section, 4th Edition. Nov. 1985.

American Backflow Prevention Association, P.O. Box 1563 Akron, Ohio 44309-1563.

Angele, Gustave *Cross-Connection and Backflow Prevention,* American Water Works Association. Supplementary Reading library Series – No. S106, New York 10016.

A Revision of The Notional Plumbing Code, ASA A40.8-1955, Report of the Public Health Service Technical Committee on Plumbing Standards. Sept. 15, 1962, Public Health Service, Washington 25, D.C.

AWWA Standard For Backflow Prevention Devices - Reduced Pressure Principle and Double Check Valve Types (C509-78), American Water Works Association, Denver, Colorado, Reaffirmed 1983. Backflow Prevention and Cross-Connection Control, AWWA Manual M14, American Water Works Association, Denver, Colorado 1966.

Backflow Prevention and Cross-Connection Control, Ohio EPA, Office of Public. Water Supply. Second Edition, Revised Mar. 15, 1977. Backflow Prevention Devices—Selection, Installation, Maintenance, and Field Testing, CSA Standard B64.10M1981. Canadian Standards Association, Dec.1981.

Backflow—The Manual of Cross-Connection Prevention in Public Water Supplies, Missouri Dept. of Natural Resources.

Canadian Plumbing Code 1980, NRCC, No. 17305, Second Printing, Issued by the Associate Committee on the National Building Code, Natural Research Council of Canada, Ottawa.

Control and Elimination of Cross-Connections, Panel Discussion, *Journal American Water Works Association,* Vol.50, No.1, 1960.

Cross-Connection Complications, *The Capital's Health,* Vol. 11, No. 9, Dec. 1953, D.C. Dept. of Public Health, Washington, D.C.

Cross-Connection Control, American Water Works Association, British Columbia Section, Second Edition, Jan.1980. *Cross-Connection Control and Backflow Prevention Device Testing,* New England Water Works Association, August 1987.

Cross-Connection Control and Backflow Prevention, Practice and Procedure Manual, Administrative Manual, City of Winnipeg, Manitoba. Third Edition, April 1980.

Cross-Connection Control, Backflow Prevention Device Tester Certification Training Course, Public Drinking Water Program, Division of Environmental Quality, Department of Natural Resources, State of Missouri.

Cross-Connection Control Manual, Division of Sanitary Engineering, Tennessee Dept. of Public Health, 1975.

Cross-Connection Control Regulation in Washington State, Washington State Dept. of Social and Health Services, Denver, Colorado, 1974. Second Edition.

Cross-Connection Control, New York State Dept. of Health, Jan.1981.

Cross-Connection Control Program, State of Utah, Oct.1985, Travis Black.

Cross-Connection Control, Water Quality Division, Colorado Department of Health. Revised March 1983. Cross-Connection Control Survey, New England Water Works Association, August 1987.

CSA Standards on Vacuum Breakers and Backflow Preventers, B64 Series 1976 Canadian Standards Association, Dec.1976.

Dawson, F. M., and Kalinske, A. A., Report on *Cross-Connections and Backsiphonage Research,* Technical Bulletin No. 1, National Association of Plumbing, Heating, Cooling Contractors, Washington, D.C.

Evaluation of Backflow Prevention Devices—A State of the Art, (N B SIR 76-1070) U.S. Environmental Protection Agency, Water Supply Division, Washington, D.C., June 1976.

Hendrickson, Howard D. *Cross-Connection Control,* Part 1 & 2, August & September 1981 issues of Reeves Journal.

How To Prevent Industrial Cross-Connection Dangers, *Water Works Engineering,* Feb. 1962. Manitoba Plumbing Code 1981, Issued by the Department of Labour and Manpower of the Province of Manitoba.

Manual of Cross-Connection Control, Dept. of Health and Hospitals, Denver, Colorado, 1977.

Manual of Cross-Connection Control, Foundation for Cross-Connection Control and Hydraulic Research, University of Southern California, 7th Editions, June 1985.

Manual of Cross-Connection Control Practices and Procedures, State of California, Health and Welfare Agency, July 1981.

Plumbing and Drainage Act Regulations, Alberta, as amended by Alberta Regulations (295/80).

Regulations Relating To Cross-Connections, excerpt from the California Administrative Code, Title 17, Public Health, 1956.

Saskatchewan Regulations 8/78, Regulations Governing Plumbing and Drainage

Solar Domestic Hot Water Systems and the Water Purveyor, American Water Works Association, Pacific Northwest Section.

Springer, E. K., and Reynolds, K. C., *Definitions and Specifications of Double Check Valve Assemblies and Reduced Pressure Principle Backflow Prevention Devices,* University of Southern California, School of Engineering Dept. 48-101, Jan. 30, 1959.

Taylor, F. B., and Skodje, M. T., Cross-Connections, *A Hazard in All Buildings, Modern Sanitation and Building Maintenance,* Vol.14, No.8, Aug. 1962.

Use of Backflow Preventers for Cross-Connection Control, Joint Committee Report, *Journal American Water Works Association,* Vol. 50, No.12, Dec. 1958.

Van Meter, R. O., Backflow Prevention Hardware, Water and Wastes Engineering, Pt. 1, Sept. 1970; Pt. 2, Oct. 1970.

Cross-Connection Survey Form

Date: _____

Name of Company, Corporation, or Business: _____

_____

Address: _____

Name of Contact: _____

Type of Use: Industrial _____   Commercial _____   Governmental _____   Other

Location of Service: _____

Size of Service: _____ Inch	Metered?	Yes ☐	No ☐
Require non-interrupted water service?		Yes ☐	No ☐
Does Boiler Feed utilize chemical additives?		Yes ☐	No ☐
Is Backflow protection incorporated?		Yes ☐	No ☐
Are air conditioning cooling towers utilized?		Yes ☐	No ☐
Is Backflow protection incorporated?		Yes ☐	No ☐
Is a Water Saver utilized on condensing lines or cooling towers?	N/A ☐	Yes ☐	No ☐
Is the make-up supply line backflow protected?		Yes ☐	No ☐
Is process water in use, and if so, is it potable supply water or "Raw" water		N/A ☐	Potable ☐
	Raw ☐	Protected ☐	Unprotected ☐
Is fire protection water separate from the potable supply?		Yes ☐	No ☐
Are Containment Devices in place?		Yes ☐	No ☐

Summary

Degree of Hazard:		High ☐	Low ☐
Type of Device recommended for containment:	RPZ ☐	DCV ☐	None ☐
Fixture Outlet protection required?		Yes ☐	No ☐

If so, where?

Backflow Prevention Device Test and Maintenance Report

To: _____
　　　(water purveyor or regulatory agency)

_____

_____

Attn: Cross-connection Control Section

The cross-connection control device detailed hereon has been tested and maintained as required by the *(rules or regulations)* of *(purveyor or regulatory agency)* and is certified to comply with these *(rules or regulations)*.

Make of device _____　　size _____

Model Number _____　　located at _____

Serial Number _____　　　　　　_____

　　　　　　　　　　　　　　　　　　　　　_____

| | Reduced Pressure Devices | | | Pressure Vacuum Breaker | |
| | Double Check Devices | | Relief Valve | Air Inlet | Check Valve |
	1st Check	2nd Check			
Initial Test	DC - Closed Tight ☐ RP - _____ psid Leaked ☐	Closed Tight ☐ Leaked ☐	Opened at _____ psid	Opened at _____ psid Did not open ☐	_____ psid Leaked ☐
Repairs and Materials Used					
Test After Repair	DC-Closed Tight RP- _____ psid	Closed Tight ☐	Opened at _____ psid	Opened at _____ psid	_____ psid

The above is certified to be true.

Firm Name _____　　Certified Tester _____

Firm Address _____　　Cert. Tester No. _____ Date _____

_____

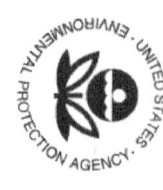

WH-550
United States
Environmental Protection
Agency
Washington, DC 20460

Official Business
Penalty for Private Use
$300

Office of Water (4606M)
EPA 816-R-03-002
www.epa.gov/safewater
February 2003